ARTHRITIS PAIN RELIEF

How to Manage Pain and Improve Mobility

Phillip J. Richmond

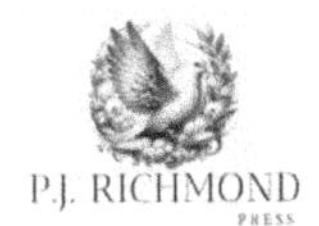

P.J. RICHMOND
PRESS

Dedication

To all the people living with arthritis, who face each day with courage and resilience. This book is for you. May you find hope, comfort, and relief in these pages.

Also By Phillip J. Richmond

Table of contents

Introduction

Arthritis is a common and chronic condition that affects millions of people around the world. It is not a single disease, but a term that covers over 100 different types of joint disorders. Arthritis causes inflammation, pain, stiffness, and damage to the joints, which can limit your mobility and function. Arthritis can affect any joint in your body, but it is more common in the hands, knees, hips, and spine.

There are many different types of arthritis, each with its own causes, symptoms, and treatments. Some of the most common types are:

- **Osteoarthritis**: This is the most common type of arthritis, which occurs when the cartilage that cushions the ends of the bones wears away, causing the bones to rub against each other. This leads to pain, swelling, and reduced motion. Osteoarthritis can result from aging, injury, obesity, or genetic factors.

- **Rheumatoid arthritis**: This is an autoimmune disease, which means that your immune system mistakenly attacks your own tissues, causing inflammation and damage to the joints and other organs. Rheumatoid arthritis can cause pain, stiffness, swelling, and deformity of the joints, as well as fatigue, fever, and weight loss. Rheumatoid arthritis can affect anyone, but it is more common in women and older adults.

- **Gout**: This is a type of arthritis that occurs when uric acid, a waste product in the blood, builds up and forms crystals in the joints, especially in the big toe. This causes sudden and severe attacks of pain, swelling, redness, and warmth. Gout can be triggered by eating certain foods, drinking alcohol, or taking certain medications.

- **Psoriatic arthritis**: This is a type of arthritis that affects some people who have psoriasis, a skin condition that causes red, scaly patches on the skin. Psoriatic arthritis can cause inflammation, pain, and stiffness in the joints, as well as skin and nail changes. Psoriatic arthritis can affect any joint, but it is more common in the fingers, toes, spine, and sacroiliac joints.

- **Lupus**: This is another autoimmune disease, which means that your immune system mistakenly attacks your own tissues, causing inflammation and damage to the joints and other organs. Lupus can cause pain, swelling, and stiffness in the joints, as well as rash, fever, fatigue, and kidney problems. Lupus can affect anyone, but it is more common in women and young adults.

These are just some of the many types of arthritis that exist. Each type of arthritis has its own characteristics, risk factors, diagnosis, and treatment. However, they all share some common symptoms and complications, such as:

- **Pain**: This is the most common and obvious symptom of arthritis. Pain can range from mild to severe, and can vary depending on the type, location, and severity of the arthritis. Pain can affect your daily activities, sleep, mood, and quality of life.

- **Swelling**: This is another common symptom of arthritis, which occurs when the joint becomes inflamed and fluid accumulates in the joint space. Swelling can cause the joint to look larger, feel warmer, and be more sensitive to touch. Swelling can also limit your range of motion and function.

- **Stiffness**: This is a common symptom of arthritis, which occurs when the joint becomes less flexible and harder to move. Stiffness can be worse in the morning or after a period of inactivity. Stiffness can make it difficult to perform simple tasks, such as opening a jar, tying your shoes, or brushing your teeth.

- **Damage**: This is a common complication of arthritis, which occurs when the joint structure and function deteriorate over time. Damage can result from the wear and tear of the cartilage and bone, the erosion of the joint capsule and ligaments, or the deformation of the joint shape. Damage can cause more pain, swelling, stiffness, and disability.

Arthritis can have a significant impact on your quality of life and mental health. Arthritis can affect your ability to work, study, socialize, and enjoy your hobbies. Arthritis can also affect your self-esteem, confidence, and body image. Arthritis can increase your risk of developing other health problems, such as cardiovascular disease, diabetes, obesity, depression, and anxiety.

The good news is that arthritis is not a hopeless condition. There are many ways to manage your pain and improve your mobility, and to live well and enjoy life with arthritis. The goals and benefits of pain relief and improved mobility are:

- To reduce your pain and discomfort, and to improve your physical and emotional well-being.
- To increase your range of motion and function, and to prevent or delay further joint damage and disability.
- To enhance your independence and autonomy, and to enable you to perform your daily activities and roles.

- To improve your social and interpersonal relationships, and to expand your opportunities and experiences.

In this book, you will learn how to achieve these goals and benefits, and how to cope with the challenges and opportunities that arthritis can bring. You will discover the best practices and strategies for managing your arthritis pain naturally and effectively, such as diet, nutrition, hydration, exercise, physical therapy, stretching, flexibility, posture, alignment, complementary and alternative therapies, stress management, emotional coping, social support, and living well and enjoying life with arthritis.

This book is based on the latest scientific evidence and research, as well as the personal stories and experiences of people who have overcome arthritis and achieved their goals and dreams. This book is designed to be informative, practical, and inspirational, and to empower you to take charge of your arthritis and your life.

Whether you have been recently diagnosed with arthritis, or you have been living with it for a long time, this book will help you to understand your condition, explore your treatment options, and apply the tips and strategies that work best for you. This book will also help you to cope with the emotional and social aspects of arthritis, and to find meaning and purpose in your life.

Arthritis does not have to define you or limit you. You can manage your pain and improve your mobility, and you can live well and enjoy life with arthritis. This book will show you how. Let's get started!

Fact:

There are over 100 different types of arthritis, with osteoarthritis and rheumatoid arthritis being the most common forms.

Chapter 1: The Role of Diet and Nutrition in Arthritis Pain Relief

Arthritis is a common condition that affects millions of people around the world. It causes pain, stiffness, swelling, and reduced mobility in the joints. Arthritis can affect any joint in the body, but it is more common in the hands, knees, hips, and spine. Arthritis is not a single disease, but a term that covers over 100 different types of joint disorders. Some of the most common types are osteoarthritis, rheumatoid arthritis, gout, and psoriatic arthritis. Each type of arthritis has different causes, symptoms, and treatments.

If you are experiencing joint pain and suspect that you have arthritis, the first step is to get a proper diagnosis from your doctor. A correct diagnosis will help you understand the type and severity of your condition, and guide you to the best treatment options for your situation.

How to get a proper diagnosis and what tests are involved

To diagnose arthritis, your doctor will ask you about your medical history, your symptoms, and your lifestyle. They will also examine your joints and look for signs of inflammation, damage, or deformity. Depending on the type of arthritis you may have, your doctor may order some tests to confirm the diagnosis and rule out other possible causes of your joint pain. Some of the common tests for arthritis are:

- **Blood tests**: These can measure the levels of certain substances in your blood, such as antibodies, inflammatory markers, uric acid, or glucose. Blood tests can help identify rheumatoid arthritis, gout, lupus, and other types of inflammatory arthritis.
- **X-rays**: These can show the structure and condition of your bones and joints. X-rays can reveal the presence and extent of joint damage, such as erosion, narrowing, or deformity. X-rays can help diagnose osteoarthritis, rheumatoid arthritis, and other types of degenerative arthritis.

- **Ultrasound**: This uses sound waves to create images of your soft tissues, such as cartilage, ligaments, tendons, and bursae. Ultrasound can detect inflammation, fluid, or damage in these structures. Ultrasound can help diagnose rheumatoid arthritis, gout, bursitis, and other types of soft tissue arthritis.

- **MRI**: This uses magnetic fields and radio waves to create detailed images of your bones and soft tissues. MRI can show the condition and integrity of your cartilage, ligaments, tendons, and nerves. MRI can help diagnose osteoarthritis, rheumatoid arthritis, psoriatic arthritis, and other types of complex arthritis.

- **Joint aspiration**: This involves inserting a needle into your joint and drawing out some fluid for analysis. Joint fluid can contain clues about the type and cause of your arthritis, such as crystals, bacteria, or blood. Joint aspiration can help diagnose gout, septic arthritis, hemarthrosis, and other types of acute arthritis.

Your doctor may order one or more of these tests, depending on your symptoms and suspected type of arthritis. The results of these tests will help your doctor make a definitive diagnosis and plan your treatment accordingly.

The conventional treatments for arthritis

Once you have a diagnosis, your doctor will discuss with you the available treatment options for your type and severity of arthritis. The main goals of arthritis treatment are to reduce pain, inflammation, and joint damage, and to improve your function and quality of life. The conventional treatments for arthritis include medications, injections, and surgery. These treatments can be used alone or in combination, depending on your condition and preferences. Here is a brief overview of each treatment option and its pros and cons.

Medications

Medications are the most common and first-line treatment for most types of arthritis. There are different kinds of medications that can help with arthritis, such as:

- **Analgesics**: These are painkillers that can relieve mild to moderate pain, but do not reduce inflammation. Examples are acetaminophen, tramadol, and opioids.

- **Nonsteroidal anti-inflammatory drugs (NSAIDs)**: These can reduce both pain and inflammation, but may cause side effects such as stomach ulcers, bleeding, kidney damage, or cardiovascular problems. Examples are ibuprofen, naproxen, and celecoxib.

- **Corticosteroids**: These are powerful anti-inflammatory drugs that can quickly reduce pain, swelling, and stiffness, but may cause side effects such as weight gain, diabetes, osteoporosis, or infections. Examples are prednisone, methylprednisolone, and dexamethasone.

- **Disease-modifying antirheumatic drugs (DMARDs)**: These are drugs that can slow down or stop the progression of inflammatory arthritis, such as rheumatoid arthritis, psoriatic arthritis, or lupus. They may take weeks or months to work, but can prevent or delay joint damage and disability.

Examples are methotrexate, sulfasalazine, and hydroxychloroquine.

- **Biologic agents**: These are a newer class of DMARDs that target specific molecules involved in the inflammatory process. They can be more effective and faster than conventional DMARDs, but may cause side effects such as infections, allergic reactions, or cancer. Examples are etanercept, infliximab, and adalimumab.

The pros of medications are that they are easy to use, widely available, and relatively affordable. They can provide significant relief from pain and inflammation, and some can even modify the course of the disease. The cons of medications are that they may not work for everyone, they may lose their effectiveness over time, and they may cause serious side effects or interactions with other drugs. You should always consult your doctor before taking any medication, and follow their instructions carefully.

Injections

Injections are another treatment option for arthritis, especially when medications are not enough or cause intolerable side effects. Injections can deliver drugs directly into the affected joint or the surrounding tissues, such as:

- **Corticosteroid injections**: These are injections of anti-inflammatory steroids that can quickly reduce pain, swelling, and stiffness in the joint. They can last for weeks or months, but may cause side effects such as joint infection, cartilage damage, or bone loss. They should not be used more than three or four times a year in the same joint.

- **Hyaluronic acid injections**: These are injections of a natural substance that lubricates and cushions the joint. They can improve the joint's function and mobility, and reduce pain and inflammation. They can last for six months or longer, but may cause side effects such as joint infection, pain, or swelling. They are mainly used for osteoarthritis of the knee.

- **Platelet-rich plasma (PRP) injections**: These are injections of your own blood that has been enriched with platelets, which are cells that promote healing and tissue regeneration. They can stimulate the growth of new cartilage and reduce pain and inflammation in the joint. They can last for a year or longer, but may cause side effects such as joint infection, pain, or swelling. They are mainly used for osteoarthritis of the knee or hip.

- **Stem cell injections**: These are injections of your own or donated stem cells, which are cells that can differentiate into various types of tissues. They can potentially repair the damaged cartilage and regenerate the joint. They are still experimental and not widely available, but may offer a long-term solution for arthritis. They may cause side effects such as joint infection, pain, or swelling. They are mainly used for osteoarthritis of the knee or hip.

The pros of injections are that they can provide more targeted and effective relief than oral medications, and they can avoid some of the systemic side effects of drugs. They can also enhance the joint's function and mobility, and some can even restore the joint's structure. The cons of injections are that they may not work for everyone, they may have limited or temporary effects, and they may cause serious side effects or complications such as joint infection, cartilage damage, or bone loss. You should always consult your doctor before getting any injection, and follow their instructions carefully.

Surgery

Surgery is the last resort treatment for arthritis, when all other options have failed or are not suitable. Surgery can involve repairing, replacing, or removing parts of the joint, such as:

- **Arthroscopy**: This is a minimally invasive procedure that involves inserting a thin tube with a camera and instruments into the joint through small incisions. The surgeon can then inspect, repair, or remove damaged tissues, such as cartilage, ligaments, or bone spurs. Arthroscopy can improve the joint's function and mobility, and reduce pain and inflammation. It can also diagnose the cause of the joint problem. It has a short recovery time and low risk of complications, but it may not be effective for severe or advanced arthritis.

- **Osteotomy**: This is a procedure that involves cutting and reshaping the bone near the joint to improve its alignment and distribution of weight. Osteotomy can relieve the pressure and pain on the worn-out part of the joint, and delay the need for joint replacement. It has a longer recovery time and higher risk of complications than arthroscopy, but it can preserve the natural joint and its function. It is mainly used for osteoarthritis of the knee or hip.

- **Arthrodesis**: This is a procedure that involves fusing two bones together to form one rigid unit. Arthrodesis can eliminate the pain and instability caused by the damaged joint, but it also sacrifices the joint's function and mobility. It has a long recovery time and high risk of complications, such as infection, nonunion, or nerve damage.

- **Arthroplasty**: This is a procedure that involves replacing the damaged joint with an artificial one made of metal, plastic, or ceramic. Arthroplasty can restore the joint's function and mobility, and eliminate pain and inflammation. It has a long recovery time and high risk of complications, such as infection, loosening, or wear and tear. It is mainly used for severe or advanced arthritis of the knee, hip, shoulder, or elbow.

The pros of surgery are that it can provide the most definitive and lasting solution for arthritis, and it can improve your quality of life significantly. The cons of surgery are that it is invasive, expensive, and risky, and it may not work for everyone or last forever. You should always consult your doctor before considering any surgery, and weigh the benefits and risks carefully.

The pros and cons of each treatment option and how to choose the best one for you

As you can see, there are many treatment options for arthritis, each with its own advantages and disadvantages. There is no one-size-fits-all solution for arthritis, and the best treatment for you depends on several factors, such as:

- **Your type and severity of arthritis**: Different types of arthritis may respond better to different treatments. For example, DMARDs and biologics are more effective for inflammatory arthritis than for degenerative arthritis. Similarly, the severity of your arthritis may determine the need and suitability of certain treatments. For example, surgery may be more appropriate for advanced arthritis than for mild or moderate arthritis.

- **Your symptoms and goals**: Your symptoms and goals may influence your preference and tolerance for certain treatments. For example, if you have severe pain and want immediate relief, you may opt for injections or surgery over medications or physical therapy. On the other hand, if you have mild pain and want to preserve your joint function and mobility, you may prefer medications or physical therapy over injections or surgery.

- **Your medical history and condition**: Your medical history and condition may affect the safety and effectiveness of certain treatments. For example, if you have a history of stomach ulcers, bleeding, or kidney problems, you may not be able to take NSAIDs or corticosteroids. Similarly, if you have an infection, cancer, or immune disorder, you may not be able to take DMARDs or biologics. You should always inform your doctor of any medical conditions or medications you have before starting any treatment.

- **Your lifestyle and preferences**: Your lifestyle and preferences may also play a role in choosing the best treatment for you. For example, if you are busy and have difficulty remembering to take pills, you may prefer injections or surgery over medications. On the other hand, if you are afraid of needles or surgery, you may prefer medications or physical therapy over injections or surgery. You should always discuss your expectations and concerns with your doctor before deciding on any treatment.

To choose the best treatment for you, you should work with your doctor and consider all the factors mentioned above. You should also do your own research and learn as much as you can about the different treatment options, their benefits and risks, and their costs and availability. You should also seek a second opinion if you are unsure or unhappy with your doctor's recommendation. Ultimately, the decision is yours, and you should choose the treatment that suits your needs and goals the best.

The latest advances and innovations in arthritis treatment

Arthritis treatment is constantly evolving and improving, thanks to the advances and innovations in medical science and technology. Some of the latest and most promising developments in arthritis treatment are:

- **Biologics**: These are a newer class of DMARDs that target specific molecules involved in the inflammatory process. They can be more effective and faster than conventional DMARDs, but may cause side effects such as infections, allergic reactions, or cancer. Examples are etanercept, infliximab, and adalimumab. Biologics are already widely used for rheumatoid arthritis, psoriatic arthritis, and other types of inflammatory arthritis, and they may also be beneficial for osteoarthritis in the future.

- **Stem cells**: These are cells that can differentiate into various types of tissues. They can potentially repair the damaged cartilage and regenerate the joint. They are still experimental and not widely available, but may offer a long-term solution for arthritis. They may cause side effects such as joint infection, pain, or swelling. They are mainly used for osteoarthritis of the knee or hip.

- **Gene therapy**: This is a technique that involves modifying the genes of the cells in the joint to alter their function or behavior. It can potentially reduce the inflammation, pain, and damage caused by arthritis, and enhance the healing and regeneration of the joint. It is still in the early stages of research and development, but may offer a novel and personalized approach for arthritis treatment. It may cause side effects such as infections, immune reactions, or cancer. It is mainly used for rheumatoid arthritis and other types of inflammatory arthritis.

These are some of the latest and most exciting developments in arthritis treatment, but they are not without challenges and limitations. They are still undergoing clinical trials and regulatory approvals, and they may not be accessible or affordable for everyone. They may also have unknown or unforeseen consequences or complications, and they may not work for everyone or last forever. You should always consult your doctor before trying any new or experimental treatment, and be aware of the potential benefits and risks involved.

The questions to ask your doctor and the things to consider before starting any treatment

Before starting any treatment for arthritis, you should ask your doctor some important questions and consider some essential things, such as:

- **What is the diagnosis and prognosis of my arthritis?**: You should understand the type and severity of your arthritis, and how it may affect your joint function and mobility, your quality of life, and your overall health. You should also know the expected course and outcome of your arthritis, and how it may change over time or with treatment.

- **What are the treatment options and goals for my arthritis?**: You should know the available treatment options for your arthritis, and how they work, how they are used, and how they may help you. You should also know the goals of the treatment, and what you can expect from it in terms of pain relief, inflammation reduction, joint function improvement, and disease modification.

- **What are the benefits and risks of each treatment option?**: You should know the advantages and disadvantages of each treatment option, and how they may affect your symptoms, your joint condition, and your overall health. You should also know the possible side effects or complications of each treatment option, and how they can be prevented or managed.

- **What are the costs and availability of each treatment option?**: You should know the expenses and insurance coverage of each treatment option, and how they may affect your budget and access to care. You should also know the availability and convenience of each treatment option, and how they may fit your schedule and lifestyle.

- **What are your recommendations and preferences for my treatment?**: You should listen to your doctor's advice and suggestions for your treatment, and understand their rationale and evidence behind them. You should also express your own preferences and concerns for your treatment, and discuss them with your doctor openly and honestly.

- **What are the alternatives or complementary therapies for my treatment?**: You should know the other options or additional therapies that may enhance or supplement your treatment, such as physical therapy, exercise, diet, supplements, acupuncture, massage, or meditation. You should also know the effectiveness and safety of these therapies, and how they may interact with your treatment.

These are some of the questions to ask and things to consider before starting any treatment for arthritis. You should always communicate with your doctor clearly and frequently, and make informed and shared decisions about your treatment. You should also monitor your response and progress with your treatment, and report any changes or problems to your doctor promptly. You should also follow your treatment plan faithfully, and adhere to your doctor's instructions and recommendations.

Arthritis is a common and complex condition that causes pain, inflammation, and damage in the joints. It can affect your function and mobility, and your quality of life. Arthritis can be diagnosed by your doctor through your history, examination, and tests. Arthritis can be treated by various options, such as medications, injections, and surgery. Each treatment option has its pros and cons, and the best one for you depends on your type and severity of arthritis, your symptoms and goals, your medical history and condition, and your lifestyle and preferences. You should work with your doctor to choose the best treatment for you, and ask questions and consider things before starting any treatment. You should also follow your treatment plan and monitor your response and progress. Arthritis can be a challenging condition, but with proper diagnosis and treatment, you can manage your pain and improve your mobility.

Chapter 2: Eating Well and Staying Hydrated for Arthritis

One of the most important factors that can influence your arthritis pain and mobility is your diet and nutrition. What you eat and drink can have a significant impact on your inflammation level, joint health, and overall well-being. By following a healthy and balanced diet, you can reduce your pain, improve your mobility, and prevent or delay further joint damage and complications.

In this chapter, you will learn how diet and nutrition can affect your arthritis, and how to make the best choices for your needs and preferences. You will discover:

- The role of diet and nutrition in reducing inflammation and pain.
- The best foods and supplements to eat and avoid for arthritis.
- The importance of hydration and how to drink enough water.

- The tips and tricks for planning and preparing healthy meals and snacks

By the end of this chapter, you will have a clear and comprehensive understanding of how diet and nutrition can help you to manage your arthritis pain and improve your mobility. You will be ready to take the next steps towards creating and following a personalized and enjoyable diet plan that works for you.

The Role of Diet and Nutrition in Reducing Inflammation and Pain

One of the main causes of arthritis pain is inflammation. Inflammation is a natural and protective response of your body to injury, infection, or irritation. However, when inflammation becomes chronic and excessive, it can damage your joints and other tissues, and cause pain, swelling, stiffness, and reduced mobility.

Diet and nutrition can play a key role in modulating your inflammation level and pain. Some foods and nutrients can trigger or worsen inflammation, while others can reduce or prevent it. By eating more anti-inflammatory foods and nutrients, and avoiding or limiting pro-inflammatory foods and nutrients, you can lower your inflammation level and pain, and improve your joint health and function.

Some of the most common anti-inflammatory foods and nutrients are:

- **Omega-3 fatty acids**: These are essential fats that your body cannot produce on its own, and that you need to obtain from your diet. Omega-3 fatty acids have anti-inflammatory properties, and can help to reduce the production of inflammatory chemicals in your body, such as prostaglandins and cytokines. Omega-3 fatty acids can also help to improve your blood flow, lower your blood pressure, and protect your heart and brain health. Some of the best sources of omega-3 fatty acids are fatty fish, such as salmon, tuna, mackerel, and sardines, as well as fish oil supplements, flaxseeds, chia seeds, walnuts, and soybeans.

- **Antioxidants**: These are substances that can protect your cells from the damage caused by free radicals, which are unstable molecules that can cause inflammation and oxidative stress. Antioxidants can help to neutralize free radicals, and prevent or repair the damage they cause to your joints and other tissues. Antioxidants can also help to boost your immune system, and prevent or fight infections. Some of the most common antioxidants are vitamins A, C, and E, as well as beta-carotene, lycopene, lutein, and flavonoids. Some of the best sources of antioxidants are fruits and vegetables, especially those that are brightly colored, such as berries, citrus fruits, tomatoes, carrots, spinach, and broccoli, as well as green tea, dark chocolate, and red wine.

- **Fiber**: This is a type of carbohydrate that your body cannot digest, and that passes through your digestive system intact. Fiber can help to reduce inflammation and pain, by lowering your blood sugar and insulin levels, improving your cholesterol and triglyceride levels, and promoting the growth of beneficial bacteria in your gut. Fiber can also help to regulate your bowel movements, prevent constipation, and lower your risk of colon cancer. Some of the best sources of fiber are whole grains, such as oats, barley, quinoa, and brown rice, as well as beans, lentils, nuts, seeds, fruits, and vegetables.

- **Spices and herbs**: These are plant-based substances that can add flavor and aroma to your food, as well as provide health benefits. Many spices and herbs have anti-inflammatory properties, and can help to reduce the production or activity of inflammatory chemicals in your body, such as prostaglandins, cytokines, and nuclear factor-kappa B. Some of the most common spices and herbs that have anti-inflammatory effects are turmeric, ginger, garlic, onion, cinnamon, clove, rosemary, thyme, oregano, and basil.

Some of the most common pro-inflammatory foods and nutrients are:

- **Saturated fats**: These are fats that are solid at room temperature, and that can increase your inflammation level and pain, by stimulating the production of inflammatory chemicals in your body, such as prostaglandins and cytokines. Saturated fats can also raise your cholesterol and triglyceride levels, and increase your risk of heart disease and stroke. Some of the main sources of saturated fats are animal products, such as red meat, poultry skin, butter, cheese, and cream, as well as coconut oil and palm oil.

- **Trans fats**: These are fats that are artificially created by adding hydrogen to liquid vegetable oils, and that can increase your inflammation level and pain, by stimulating the production of inflammatory chemicals in your body, such as prostaglandins and cytokines. Trans fats can also raise your cholesterol and triglyceride levels, and increase your risk of heart disease and stroke. Some of the main sources of trans fats are processed and fried foods, such as pastries, cakes, cookies, chips, and donuts, as well as margarine and shortening.

- **Refined carbohydrates**: These are carbohydrates that have been stripped of their fiber, vitamins, minerals, and phytochemicals, and that can increase your inflammation level and pain, by raising your blood sugar and insulin levels, and triggering the release of inflammatory chemicals in your body, such as prostaglandins and cytokines. Refined carbohydrates can also increase your appetite, weight, and fat storage, and lower your energy and mood. Some of the main sources of refined carbohydrates are white bread, white rice, white pasta, white flour, sugar, and corn syrup.

- **Added sugars**: These are sugars that are added to foods and drinks during processing or preparation, and that can increase your inflammation level and pain, by raising your blood sugar and insulin levels, and triggering the release of inflammatory chemicals in your body, such as prostaglandins and cytokines. Added sugars can also increase your appetite, weight, and fat storage, and lower your energy and mood. Some of the main sources of added sugars are soft drinks, fruit juices, candy, chocolate, ice cream, and desserts, as well as sauces, dressings, and condiments.

- **Alcohol**: This is a substance that can increase your inflammation level and pain, by interfering with your liver function, and increasing the production of inflammatory chemicals in your body, such as prostaglandins and cytokines. Alcohol can also dehydrate you, impair your judgment, and increase your risk of liver disease, pancreatitis, and cancer. Some of the main sources of alcohol are beer, wine, liquor, and cocktails.

These are some of the common foods and nutrients that can affect your inflammation level and pain. However, there may be other foods and nutrients that can trigger or worsen your inflammation and pain, depending on your individual sensitivity and reaction. Therefore, it is important to pay attention to how your body responds to different foods and nutrients, and to identify and avoid or limit those that cause you problems. You can do this by keeping a food diary, and recording what you eat and drink, and how you feel afterwards. You can also consult your doctor or a nutritionist for advice and guidance.

Best Foods and Supplements to Eat and Avoid for Arthritis

Based on the role of diet and nutrition in reducing inflammation and pain, you can create a list of the best foods and supplements to eat and avoid for arthritis. Here is a possible list, based on the general recommendations and guidelines for a healthy and balanced diet, as well as the specific needs and preferences of people with arthritis. However, you can modify this list according to your individual situation and goals, and consult your doctor or a nutritionist for more information and support.

The best foods and supplements to eat for arthritis are:

- Fatty fish, such as salmon, tuna, mackerel, and sardines, or fish oil supplements, for omega-3 fatty acids.
- Fruits and vegetables, especially those that are brightly colored, such as berries, citrus fruits,

tomatoes, carrots, spinach, and broccoli, for antioxidants.

- Whole grains, such as oats, barley, quinoa, and brown rice, for fiber.
- Beans, lentils, nuts, seeds, soybeans, and tofu, for protein, fiber, and phytochemicals.
- Spices and herbs, such as turmeric, ginger, garlic, onion, cinnamon, clove, rosemary, thyme, oregano, and basil, for anti-inflammatory effects.
- Green tea, dark chocolate, and red wine, in moderation, for antioxidants and flavonoids.
- Water, for hydration and detoxification

The best foods and supplements to avoid or limit for arthritis are:

- Red meat, poultry skin, butter, cheese, cream, coconut oil, and palm oil, for saturated fats.
- Processed and fried foods, such as pastries, cakes, cookies, chips, and donuts, as well as margarine and shortening, for trans fats.
- White bread, white rice, white pasta, white flour, sugar, and corn syrup, for refined carbohydrates.

- Soft drinks, fruit juices, candy, chocolate, ice cream, and desserts, as well as sauces, dressings, and condiments, for added sugars.
- Beer, wine, liquor, and cocktails, for alcohol.
- Any foods or nutrients that you are allergic, intolerant, or sensitive to, or that trigger or worsen your inflammation and pain.

These are some of the general guidelines for the best foods and supplements to eat and avoid for arthritis. However, you may need to adjust your diet and nutrition according to your specific type of arthritis, your medication use, your health status, and your personal preferences. For example, if you have gout, you may need to limit your intake of purine-rich foods, such as organ meats, shellfish, and beer, as they can increase your uric acid level and trigger gout attacks. If you are taking blood thinners, such as warfarin, you may need to monitor your intake of vitamin K-rich foods, such as leafy greens, broccoli, and soybeans, as they can interfere with your medication effectiveness. If you have diabetes, you may need to control your carbohydrate intake and monitor your blood sugar level. If you have food allergies, intolerances, or sensitivities, you may need to avoid or limit the foods or nutrients that cause you problems, such as gluten, dairy, eggs, nuts, or nightshades.

Therefore, it is important to consult your doctor or a nutritionist before making any changes to your diet and nutrition, and to follow their advice and recommendations. They can help you to create a personalized and balanced diet plan that meets your nutritional needs and goals, and that suits your taste and lifestyle.

Importance of Hydration and How to Drink Enough Water

Another important factor that can influence your arthritis pain and mobility is your hydration level. Hydration is the state of having enough water in your body to perform its functions properly. Water is essential for your body, as it makes up about 60% of your body weight, and it is involved in many processes, such as:

- Transporting nutrients and oxygen to your cells.
- Removing waste products and toxins from your body.

- Regulating your body temperature and blood pressure.
- Lubricating your joints and cushioning your organs.
- Maintaining your skin health and appearance.
- Supporting your brain function and mood

Hydration can play a key role in modulating your arthritis pain and mobility. Some of the benefits of hydration for arthritis are:

- **Reducing inflammation and pain**: Water can help to flush out the inflammatory chemicals and waste products from your joints and other tissues, and to reduce the friction and pressure in your joints. Water can also help to prevent or relieve headaches, muscle cramps, and fatigue, which can worsen your pain and discomfort.

- **Improving mobility and function**: Water can help to lubricate your joints and improve your range of motion and flexibility. Water can also help to prevent or treat dehydration, which can cause stiffness, weakness, and dizziness, and impair your balance and coordination.

- **Preventing or delaying joint damage and complications**: Water can help to nourish your cartilage and bone, and to prevent or slow down the degeneration and erosion of your joint structure and function. Water can also help to prevent or treat kidney stones, urinary tract infections, and constipation, which can be caused or aggravated by arthritis or its medications.

The amount of water that you need to drink to stay hydrated depends on various factors, such as your age, weight, activity level, climate, health status, and medication use. However, a general guideline is to drink about 8 glasses of water per day, or about 2 liters. You may need to drink more or less water depending on your individual situation and needs. You can check your hydration level by looking at the color and volume of your urine. If your urine is clear or pale yellow, and you urinate frequently and in large amounts, you are likely well hydrated. If your urine is dark yellow, brown, or red, and you urinate infrequently and in small amounts, you are likely dehydrated.

Some of the tips and tricks for drinking enough water and staying hydrated are:

- Drink water throughout the day, and not just when you are thirsty. Thirst is a sign that you are already dehydrated, and you need to drink water to replenish your fluid loss.

- Drink water before, during, and after exercise, especially if you sweat a lot or exercise in hot or humid conditions. You can lose a lot of water and electrolytes through sweat, and you need to replace them to prevent dehydration and electrolyte imbalance.

- Drink water before, during, and after meals, especially if you eat salty, spicy, or processed foods. These foods can increase your water and sodium intake, and you need to balance them with water to prevent water retention and high blood pressure.

- Drink water with lemon, lime, cucumber, mint, or berries, to add some flavor and nutrients to your water. You can also drink herbal teas, such as chamomile, peppermint, or ginger, to hydrate yourself and to enjoy some health benefits.

However, avoid or limit caffeinated drinks, such as coffee, black tea, or energy drinks, as they can dehydrate you and increase your inflammation and pain. Also, avoid or limit alcoholic drinks, such as beer, wine, or liquor, as they can dehydrate you and increase your inflammation and pain.

- Carry a water bottle with you wherever you go, and refill it whenever you can. You can also set reminders or alarms on your phone or computer, to remind you to drink water regularly. You can also use apps or trackers, to monitor your water intake and hydration level.

These are some of the tips and tricks for drinking enough water and staying hydrated. However, you may need to adjust your water intake and hydration level according to your specific situation and goals, and consult your doctor or a nutritionist for more information and support. They can help you to determine the optimal amount and type of water that you need to drink, and to avoid or treat any problems related to hydration, such as dehydration, water intoxication, or electrolyte imbalance.

Tips and Tricks for Planning and Preparing Healthy Meals and Snacks

One of the challenges that you may face when following a healthy and balanced diet for arthritis is planning and preparing your meals and snacks. You may find it difficult to plan and prepare your meals and snacks, due to various reasons, such as:

- Lack of time, energy, or motivation.
- Lack of knowledge, skills, or resources.
- Lack of variety, taste, or appeal.
- Lack of support, guidance, or feedback.

However, planning and preparing your meals and snacks can be easier and more enjoyable, if you follow some tips and tricks, such as:

1. **Plan ahead**: Planning your meals and snacks ahead of time can help you to save time, money, and effort, and to avoid stress, temptation, and impulse. You can plan your meals and snacks for the week, or for the day, depending on your preference and convenience. You can use a calendar, a planner, a notebook, or an app, to write down your meal and

snack ideas, and to create your shopping list. You can also use online tools, such as websites, blogs, or podcasts, to find recipes, tips, and inspiration for your meals and snacks.

2. **Shop smart**: Shopping smart can help you to buy the best foods and supplements for your arthritis, and to avoid the worst ones. You can shop smart by following these guidelines:

- Shop with a list, and stick to it. This can help you to buy only what you need, and to avoid buying what you don't need or want.

- Shop when you are not hungry, thirsty, or tired. This can help you to avoid buying unhealthy or unnecessary foods and drinks, due to hunger, thirst, or fatigue.

- Shop around the perimeter of the store, and avoid the middle aisles. This can help you to buy more fresh and natural foods, such as fruits, vegetables, fish, and meat, and to avoid more processed and packaged foods, such as chips, cookies, and soda.

- Shop for quality, not quantity. This can help you to buy more nutrient-dense and satisfying foods, such as whole grains, beans, nuts, and seeds, and to avoid more calorie-dense and empty foods, such as white bread, sugar, and corn syrup.

- Shop for variety, not monotony. This can help you to buy more diverse and colorful foods, such as berries, tomatoes, carrots, spinach, and broccoli, and to avoid more bland and boring foods, such as white rice, white pasta, white flour, and cheese.

3. **Cook smart**: Cooking smart can help you to prepare your meals and snacks in a way that preserves and enhances their nutritional value, flavor, and appeal. You can cook smart by following these guidelines:

- Cook with healthy oils, such as olive, canola, or avocado oil, and avoid or limit unhealthy oils, such as butter, coconut, or palm oil. This can help you to reduce your intake of saturated fats, and to increase your intake of omega-3 fatty acids.

- Cook with low or medium heat, and avoid or limit high heat. This can help you to prevent or reduce the formation of harmful substances, such as advanced glycation end products (AGEs), which can increase your inflammation and pain.

- Cook with water, broth, or wine, and avoid or limit oil, cream, or cheese. This can help you to reduce your intake of calories, fat, and sodium, and to increase your intake of water, antioxidants, and phytochemicals.

- Cook with spices and herbs, such as turmeric, ginger, garlic, onion, cinnamon, clove, rosemary, thyme, oregano, and basil, and avoid or limit salt, sugar, or artificial flavors. This can help you to enhance the flavor and aroma of your food, and to increase your intake of anti-inflammatory substances.

- Cook with fresh and natural ingredients, and avoid or limit processed and packaged foods. This can help you to reduce your intake of additives, preservatives, and chemicals, which can increase your inflammation and pain.

4. **Prepare in advance**: Preparing your meals and snacks in advance can help you to save time, energy, and effort, and to avoid stress, temptation, and impulse. You can prepare your meals and snacks in advance by following these tips:

- *Batch cook*: This means cooking large quantities of food at once, and storing them in the fridge or freezer for later use. You can batch cook your main dishes, such as soups, stews, casseroles, or curries, and reheat them when you need them. You can also batch cook your side dishes, such as rice, pasta, or quinoa, and mix them with different sauces, vegetables, or proteins. You can also batch cook your snacks, such as muffins, granola bars, or cookies, and store them in airtight containers or bags.

- *Chop and store*: This means chopping and storing your fruits and vegetables in the fridge or freezer for later use. You can chop and store your fruits and vegetables for your salads, smoothies, juices, or snacks, and add them to your dishes when you need them. You can also chop and store your herbs and spices, such as garlic, onion, ginger, or cilantro, and use them to flavor your food when you need them.

- *Portion and pack*: This means portioning and packing your meals and snacks in individual containers or bags, and storing them in the fridge or freezer for later use. You can portion and pack your meals and snacks for your breakfast, lunch, dinner, or snacks, and grab them when you need them. You can also portion and pack your supplements, such as vitamins, minerals, or omega-3s, and take them when you need them.

Examples and Recipes of Arthritis-Friendly Dishes and Drinks

One of the joys of following a healthy and balanced diet for arthritis is enjoying the delicious and nutritious dishes and drinks that you can make and consume. There are many examples and recipes of arthritis-friendly dishes and drinks that you can find online, in books, or in magazines, or that you can create yourself, based on your taste and creativity. Here are some examples and recipes of arthritis-friendly dishes and drinks that you can try and enjoy:

1. **Breakfast**: Oatmeal with berries and nuts. This is a simple and satisfying breakfast that can provide you with fiber, antioxidants, and omega-3s. To make it, you need:

- 1/2 cup of rolled oats
- 1 cup of water or milk of your choice
- A pinch of salt
- A handful of fresh or frozen berries, such as blueberries, raspberries, or strawberries
- A handful of chopped nuts, such as walnuts, almonds, or pistachios
- A drizzle of honey or maple syrup, if desired

To make it, you need to:
- In a small pot, bring the water or milk and salt to a boil over medium-high heat.

- Add the oats and reduce the heat to low. Simmer for about 15 minutes, stirring occasionally, until the oats are soft and creamy.

- Transfer the oatmeal to a bowl and top with the berries and nuts. Drizzle with honey or maple syrup, if desired. Enjoy!

2. **Lunch**: Salmon salad with quinoa and greens. This is a light and refreshing lunch that can provide you with protein, omega-3s, and antioxidants. To make it, you need:

- 1/4 cup of quinoa

- 1/2 cup of water or broth of your choice

- A pinch of salt

- 1 (4-ounce) salmon fillet

- 1 tablespoon of olive oil

- Salt and pepper, to taste

- 2 cups of mixed greens, such as spinach, kale, or arugula

- 1/4 cup of cherry tomatoes, halved

- 2 tablespoons of lemon juice

- 1 teaspoon of honey

- 1 teaspoon of dijon mustard

- 2 tablespoons of chopped fresh parsley

To make it, you need to:

- In a small pot, bring the water or broth and salt to a boil over high heat. Add the quinoa and reduce the heat to low. Cover and simmer for about 15 minutes, or until the quinoa is fluffy and the liquid is absorbed. Fluff with a fork and set aside.

- In a small skillet, heat the olive oil over medium-high heat. Season the salmon with salt and pepper, and place it skin-side down in the skillet. Cook for about 10 minutes, flipping once, or until the salmon is cooked through and flakes easily with a fork. Transfer to a plate and break into bite-sized pieces.

- In a large bowl, toss the greens and tomatoes with the lemon juice, honey, mustard, and parsley. Season with salt and pepper, to taste.

- To serve, divide the quinoa among two plates, and top with the salmon and the salad. Enjoy!

3. **Dinner**: Chicken and vegetable curry with brown rice. This is a warm and comforting dinner that can provide you with protein, fiber, and anti-inflammatory spices. To make it, you need:

- 1 cup of brown rice
- 2 cups of water or broth of your choice
- A pinch of salt
- 1 tablespoon of coconut oil
- 1 onion, chopped
- 2 cloves of garlic, minced
- 1 tablespoon of grated ginger
- 2 teaspoons of curry powder
- 1 teaspoon of turmeric
- 1/2 teaspoon of cumin
- 1/4 teaspoon of cinnamon
- 1/4 teaspoon of salt
- 1 (14-ounce) can of coconut milk
- 1 (14-ounce) can of diced tomatoes
- 1 pound of boneless, skinless chicken breasts, cut into bite-sized pieces
- 2 cups of chopped vegetables of your choice, such as carrots, potatoes, cauliflower, or broccoli

- 2 tablespoons of chopped fresh cilantro

To make it, you need to:

- In a medium pot, bring the water or broth and salt to a boil over high heat. Add the rice and reduce the heat to low. Cover and simmer for about 40 minutes, or until the rice is tender and the liquid is absorbed. Fluff with a fork and set aside.

- In a large skillet, heat the coconut oil over medium-high heat. Add the onion, garlic, ginger, curry powder, turmeric, cumin, cinnamon, and salt, and cook for about 10 minutes, stirring occasionally, until the onion is soft and the spices are fragrant.

- Add the coconut milk and tomatoes, and bring to a boil. Reduce the heat and simmer for about 15 minutes, stirring occasionally, until the sauce is slightly thickened.

- Add the chicken and vegetables, and bring to a boil. Reduce the heat and simmer for about 20 minutes, or until the chicken is cooked through and the vegetables are tender.

- Stir in the cilantro and season with salt and pepper, to taste.
- To serve, divide the rice among four plates, and spoon the curry over the rice. Enjoy!

4. **Snack**: Apple and peanut butter. This is a simple and satisfying snack that can provide you with fiber, protein, and healthy fats. To make it, you need:
- 1 apple, sliced
- 2 tablespoons of natural peanut butter

To make it, you just need to:
- Spread the peanut butter over the apple slices. Enjoy!

5. **Drink**: Ginger and lemon tea. This is a soothing and refreshing drink that can provide you with hydration, antioxidants, and anti-inflammatory substances. To make it, you need:
- 4 cups of water
- 1/4 cup of fresh ginger, peeled and sliced
- 1/4 cup of fresh lemon juice

- 2 tablespoons of honey, or to taste

To make it, you need to:
- In a small pot, bring the water and ginger to a boil over high heat. Reduce the heat and simmer for about 15 minutes, or until the ginger is soft and the water is infused with its flavor.
- Strain the ginger and water into a large pitcher. Stir in the lemon juice and honey, and adjust the sweetness to your liking.
- To serve, pour the tea into mugs and enjoy hot, or refrigerate and enjoy cold.

These are some examples and recipes of arthritis-friendly dishes and drinks that you can try and enjoy. However, there are many more examples and recipes that you can find online, in books, or in magazines, or that you can create yourself, based on your taste and creativity. The key is to choose foods and drinks that are healthy, balanced, and enjoyable, and that suit your needs and preferences.

Arthritis is not just a condition of the elderly; it can affect people of all ages, including children (juvenile arthritis).

Chapter 3: Exercising and Moving More for Arthritis

Arthritis can make it hard to move and exercise, but staying active is one of the best things you can do for your condition. Exercise and physical therapy can help you strengthen your joints and muscles, reduce your pain and inflammation, improve your function and mobility, and enhance your quality of life.

In this chapter, you will learn about the benefits of exercise and physical therapy for arthritis, the best types and frequency of exercise for arthritis, the tips and precautions for exercising safely and avoiding injury, the examples and routines of arthritis-friendly exercises and activities, and the ways to track and measure your progress and results.

The benefits of exercise and physical therapy for strengthening your joints and muscles

Exercise and physical therapy are essential components of arthritis treatment and management. They can provide many benefits for your joints and muscles, such as:

- **Strengthening**: Exercise and physical therapy can help you build and maintain your muscle mass, which can support and protect your joints. Stronger muscles can also improve your balance and stability, and prevent falls and injuries. Physical therapy can also teach you how to use your joints and muscles properly, and correct any faulty movements or postures that may cause pain or damage.

- **Flexibility**: Exercise and physical therapy can help you increase and preserve your range of motion, which is the ability of your joints to move in different directions. Flexible joints can allow you to perform your daily activities more easily and comfortably, and prevent stiffness and deformity. Physical therapy can also provide you with stretching exercises and manual techniques, such as massage or manipulation, to loosen and relax your tight or tense muscles and tendons.

- **Endurance**: Exercise and physical therapy can help you improve and maintain your cardiovascular fitness, which is the ability of your heart and lungs to deliver oxygen and nutrients to your muscles and tissues. Endurance can help you cope with fatigue and stress, and improve your energy and mood. Physical therapy can also monitor and adjust your exercise intensity and duration, and provide you with aerobic exercises, such as walking, cycling, or swimming, to boost your endurance.

- **Pain relief**: Exercise and physical therapy can help you reduce and manage your pain, which is the most common and bothersome symptom of arthritis. Exercise can release natural painkillers, such as endorphins, in your body, and block the pain signals from reaching your brain. Physical therapy can also apply heat, cold, ultrasound, electrical stimulation, or acupuncture to your affected joints and muscles, to ease your pain and inflammation.

- **Function and mobility**: Exercise and physical therapy can help you improve and maintain your function and mobility, which are the abilities to perform your daily tasks and move around. Exercise can improve your strength, flexibility, and endurance, which can enable you to do more things and go more places. Physical therapy can also assess and address your functional limitations and mobility impairments, and provide you with assistive devices, such as braces, splints, or walkers, to improve your function and mobility.

These are some of the benefits of exercise and physical therapy for strengthening your joints and muscles. By exercising and moving more, you can not only improve your physical health, but also your mental and emotional well-being. Exercise and physical therapy can also help you prevent or delay the progression of arthritis, and reduce the need for medications or surgery.

The best types and frequency of exercise for arthritis

Not all exercises are suitable or beneficial for arthritis. Some exercises may be too strenuous or stressful for your joints, and may worsen your pain or damage. You should choose the types and frequency of exercise that are appropriate and safe for your condition and goals.

The best types of exercise for arthritis are:

- **Low-impact aerobic exercises**: These are exercises that raise your heart rate and improve your endurance, without putting too much pressure or shock on your joints. Examples are walking, cycling, swimming, water aerobics, or elliptical training. Low-impact aerobic exercises can help you burn calories, lose weight, and reduce the load on your joints. They can also improve your cardiovascular health, mood, and energy. You should aim for at least 150 minutes of moderate-intensity or 75 minutes of vigorous-intensity low-impact aerobic exercises per week, or a combination of both.

- **Strength training exercises**: These are exercises that use resistance, such as weights, bands, or your own body weight, to build and maintain your muscle strength. Examples are lifting, pushing, pulling, or squatting. Strength training exercises can help you support and protect your joints, and improve your balance and stability. They can also prevent or slow down the loss of bone density and muscle mass that can occur with arthritis and aging. You should aim for at least two sessions of strength training exercises per week, targeting all the major muscle groups of your body.

- **Flexibility exercises**: These are exercises that stretch and lengthen your muscles and tendons, and increase your range of motion. Examples are bending, twisting, reaching, or yoga. Flexibility exercises can help you loosen and relax your tight or tense muscles and tendons, and prevent stiffness and deformity. They can also improve your posture and alignment, and reduce the risk of injury. You should aim for at least one session of flexibility

exercises per day, preferably after a warm-up or a
workout.

- **Balance exercises**: These are exercises that
challenge and improve your balance and
coordination, and prevent falls and injuries.
Examples are standing on one leg, walking
heel-to-toe, or tai chi. Balance exercises can help
you strengthen your core and stabilizer muscles, and
improve your confidence and mobility. They can
also reduce the fear of falling and the anxiety that
can accompany arthritis. You should aim for at least
three sessions of balance exercises per week,
preferably in a safe and supervised environment.

These are the best types of exercise for arthritis, but they
are not the only ones. You can also try other forms of
physical activity that you enjoy and that suit your abilities
and preferences, such as dancing, gardening, golfing, or
bowling. The key is to find something that you like and that
you can do regularly and safely.

The frequency of exercise for arthritis depends on your condition and goals, but in general, you should aim for at least 30 minutes of moderate-intensity physical activity per day, or at least 150 minutes per week. You can break up your exercise into smaller sessions of 10 minutes or more, as long as you accumulate the recommended amount. You can also vary the intensity and duration of your exercise, depending on how you feel and what you want to achieve. You should always listen to your body and adjust your exercise accordingly.

Tips and precautions for exercising safely and avoiding injury

Exercise can be beneficial for arthritis, but it can also be harmful if done incorrectly or excessively. You should follow some tips and precautions to exercise safely and avoid injury, such as:

- **Consult your doctor and physical therapist before starting any exercise program**: They can assess your condition and fitness level, and recommend the best types and frequency of exercise for you. They can also teach you how to perform the exercises correctly and safely, and provide you with a personalized exercise plan and guidance.

- **Warm up and cool down before and after each exercise session**: Warming up can prepare your joints and muscles for the exercise, and reduce the risk of injury. Cooling down can relax your joints and muscles after the exercise, and prevent soreness and stiffness. You can warm up and cool down by doing some gentle movements, such as walking, cycling, or stretching, for 5 to 10 minutes.

- **Start slowly and gradually increase your exercise intensity and duration**: You should not overdo or rush your exercise, as this can cause pain, inflammation, or damage to your joints and muscles. You should start with low-intensity and short-duration exercises, and gradually increase them as you get stronger and more comfortable. You should also vary your exercise routine, and avoid doing the same exercises every day, to prevent boredom and overuse injuries.

- **Listen to your body and respect your limits**: You should pay attention to how you feel during and after the exercise, and adjust your exercise accordingly. You should stop or reduce your exercise if you experience any pain, swelling, redness, or heat in your joints, or any unusual or severe symptoms, such as chest pain, shortness of breath, or dizziness. You should also rest and recover between your exercise sessions, and allow your joints and muscles to heal and repair.

- **Use proper equipment and techniques**: You should use appropriate and comfortable shoes, clothing, and accessories for your exercise, and make sure they fit well and are in good condition. You should also use proper equipment and techniques for your exercise, and follow the instructions and recommendations of your doctor and physical therapist. You should avoid any equipment or techniques that may cause stress or injury to your joints and muscles, such as high-impact, twisting, or jerking movements.

- **Seek professional help and advice if you have any questions or concerns**: You should not hesitate to contact your doctor or physical therapist if you have any questions or concerns about your exercise program, or if you encounter any problems or difficulties with your exercise. They can help you solve any issues and provide you with support and encouragement.

These are some of the tips and precautions for exercising safely and avoiding injury. By following them, you can make your exercise experience more enjoyable and rewarding, and prevent any harm or complications.

Examples and routines of arthritis-friendly exercises and activities

To help you get started and inspired, here are some examples and routines of arthritis-friendly exercises and activities that you can try. You can modify them according to your condition and goals, and consult your doctor and physical therapist before doing them.

<u>**Low-impact aerobic exercises**</u>

1. **Walking**: Walking is one of the simplest and most accessible low-impact aerobic exercises for arthritis. It can improve your endurance, cardiovascular health, and mood, and reduce your weight and joint load. You can walk anywhere and anytime, indoors or outdoors, alone or with others. You can start with 10 minutes of walking per day, and gradually increase to 30 minutes or more, at least three times per week. You can also vary your walking speed, distance, and terrain, to challenge yourself and avoid boredom. You should wear comfortable and supportive shoes, and warm up and cool down before and after each walking session.

2. **Cycling**: Cycling is another low-impact aerobic exercise that can benefit your arthritis. It can strengthen your leg muscles, improve your endurance and cardiovascular health, and reduce your weight and joint load. You can cycle on a stationary bike or a regular bike, indoors or outdoors, alone or with others. You can start with 10

minutes of cycling per day, and gradually increase to 30 minutes or more, at least three times per week. You can also vary your cycling speed, resistance, and route, to challenge yourself and avoid boredom. You should adjust your bike seat and handlebars to fit your height and posture, and wear a helmet and other protective gear if cycling outdoors.

3. **Swimming**: Swimming is one of the best low-impact aerobic exercises for arthritis. It can work your whole body, improve your endurance and cardiovascular health, and reduce your weight and joint load. Swimming can also provide a soothing and relaxing effect for your joints and muscles, and reduce your pain and inflammation. You can swim in a pool or a natural body of water, indoors or outdoors, alone or with others. You can start with 10 minutes of swimming per day, and gradually increase to 30 minutes or more, at least three times per week. You can also vary your swimming stroke, speed, and distance, to challenge yourself and avoid boredom. You should choose a water temperature

that is comfortable and not too hot or cold, and wear a swimsuit and goggles that fit well and are in good condition.

These are some of the examples and routines of low-impact aerobic exercises for arthritis, but they are not the only ones. You can also try other forms of low-impact aerobic exercises, such as water aerobics, elliptical training, or rowing, as long as they are suitable and safe for you.

<u>Strength training exercises</u>

1. **Lifting**: Lifting is a strength training exercise that can help you build and maintain your muscle strength, especially in your upper body. It can also improve your posture and alignment, and prevent or slow down the loss of bone density and muscle mass. You can lift weights, such as dumbbells, kettlebells, or barbells, or use machines, such as cable pulleys, or resistance bands, or use your own body weight, such as push-ups, pull-ups, or planks. You can start with light weights or low resistance, and gradually increase them as you get stronger. You can also vary your lifting exercises, such as

biceps curls, triceps extensions, shoulder presses, or chest presses, to target different muscle groups. You should aim for at least two sessions of lifting exercises per week, doing 8 to 12 repetitions of each exercise, for 2 to 3 sets. You should rest for at least one minute between each set, and for at least one day between each session. You should use proper form and technique, and avoid holding your breath or straining your joints or muscles.

2. **Pushing**: Pushing is a strength training exercise that can help you build and maintain your muscle strength, especially in your chest, shoulders, and arms. It can also improve your posture and alignment, and prevent or slow down the loss of bone density and muscle mass. You can push against a wall, a door, a bench, or the floor, or use weights, such as dumbbells, kettlebells, or barbells, or machines, such as chest press or shoulder press, or resistance bands, or use your own body weight, such as push-ups, dips, or handstands. You can start with light resistance or low difficulty, and gradually

increase them as you get stronger. You can also vary your pushing exercises, such as incline, decline, or flat push-ups, or narrow, wide, or neutral grip push-ups, to target different muscle groups. You should aim for at least two sessions of pushing exercises per week, doing 8 to 12 repetitions of each exercise, for 2 to 3 sets. You should rest for at least one minute between each set, and for at least one day between each session. You should use proper form and technique, and avoid holding your breath or straining your joints or muscles.

3. **Pulling**: Pulling is a strength training exercise that can help you build and maintain your muscle strength, especially in your back, shoulders, and arms. It can also improve your posture and alignment, and prevent or slow down the loss of bone density and muscle mass. You can pull on a rope, a towel, a band, or the floor, or use weights, such as dumbbells, kettlebells, or barbells, or machines, such as lat pulldown or rowing, or resistance bands, or use your own body weight,

such as pull-ups, chin-ups, or rows. You can start with light resistance or low difficulty, and gradually increase them as you get stronger. You can also vary your pulling exercises, such as overhand, underhand, or neutral grip pull-ups, or wide, narrow, or reverse grip rows, to target different muscle groups. You should aim for at least two sessions of pulling exercises per week, doing 8 to 12 repetitions of each exercise, for 2 to 3 sets. You should rest for at least one minute between each set, and for at least one day between each session. You should use proper form and technique, and avoid holding your breath or straining your joints or muscles.

These are some of the examples and routines of strength training exercises for arthritis, but they are not the only ones. You can also try other forms of strength training exercises, such as squats, lunges, or deadlifts, as long as they are suitable and safe for you.

1. **Bending**: Bending is a flexibility exercise that can help you stretch and lengthen your muscles and tendons, and increase your range of motion, especially in your spine, hips, and knees. It can also improve your posture and alignment, and prevent stiffness and deformity. You can bend forward, backward, sideways, or diagonally, or use props, such as a chair, a ball, or a towel, to assist or deepen your bends. You can start with gentle and shallow bends, and gradually increase them as you get more flexible. You can also vary your bending exercises, such as toe touches, back extensions, side bends, or twists, to target different muscle groups. You should aim for at least one session of bending exercises per day, preferably after a warm-up or a workout, holding each bend for 10 to 30 seconds, and repeating 2 to 4 times. You should use proper form and technique, and avoid bouncing, jerking, or forcing your bends.

2. **Twisting**: Twisting is a flexibility exercise that can help you stretch and lengthen your muscles and tendons, and increase your range of motion, especially in your spine, shoulders, and neck. It can also improve your posture and alignment, and prevent stiffness and deformity. You can twist your upper body, your lower body, or both, or use props, such as a chair, a ball, or a towel, to assist or deepen your twists. You can start with gentle and shallow twists, and gradually increase them as you get more flexible. You can also vary your twisting exercises, such as neck rotations, shoulder rolls, spine twists, or leg crosses, to target different muscle groups. You should aim for at least one session of twisting exercises per day, preferably after a warm-up or a workout, holding each twist for 10 to 30 seconds, and repeating 2 to 4 times. You should use proper form and technique, and avoid bouncing, jerking, or forcing your twists.

3. **Reaching**: Reaching is a flexibility exercise that can help you stretch and lengthen your muscles and

tendons, and increase your range of motion, especially in your arms, chest, and back. It can also improve your posture and alignment, and prevent stiffness and deformity. You can reach your arms overhead, to the sides, to the front, or to the back, or use props, such as a wall, a door, or a towel, to assist or deepen your reaches. You can start with gentle and shallow reaches, and gradually increase them as you get more flexible. You can also vary your reaching exercises, such as arm circles, chest openers, back squeezes, or shoulder stretches, to target different muscle groups. You should aim for at least one session of reaching exercises per day, preferably after a warm-up or a workout, holding each reach for 10 to 30 seconds, and repeating 2 to 4 times. You should use proper form and technique, and avoid bouncing, jerking, or forcing your reaches.

These are some of the examples and routines of flexibility exercises for arthritis, but they are not the only ones. You can also try other forms of flexibility exercises, such as yoga, pilates, or tai chi, as long as they are suitable and safe for you.

Balance exercises

1. **Standing**: Standing is a balance exercise that can help you strengthen your core and stabilizer muscles, and improve your balance and coordination, and prevent falls and injuries. It can also improve your posture and alignment, and reduce the fear of falling and the anxiety that can accompany arthritis. You can stand on one leg, on your toes, on your heels, or on an unstable surface, such as a pillow, a foam pad, or a wobble board. You can start with easy and stable standing positions, and gradually increase them as you get more confident and balanced. You can also vary your standing exercises, such as lifting your arms, closing your eyes, or turning your head, to challenge yourself and avoid boredom. You should aim for at least three sessions of standing exercises per week, preferably in a safe and supervised environment, holding each position for 10 to 30

seconds, and repeating 2 to 4 times. You should use proper form and technique, and avoid holding your breath or tensing your muscles.

2. **Walking**: Walking is another balance exercise that can help you strengthen your core and stabilizer muscles, and improve your balance and coordination, and prevent falls and injuries. It can also improve your endurance and cardiovascular health, and enhance your mood and energy. You can walk on a straight line, a curved line, or a zigzag line, or on an uneven or slippery surface, such as grass, sand, or ice. You can start with easy and smooth walking paths, and gradually increase them as you get more confident and balanced. You can also vary your walking exercises, such as changing your speed, direction, or stride length, to challenge yourself and avoid boredom. You should aim for at least three sessions of walking exercises per week, preferably in a safe and supervised environment, walking for 10 to 30 minutes, and repeating 2 to 4 times. You should use proper form and technique,

and avoid holding your breath or tensing your muscles.

3. **Tai chi**: Tai chi is a form of balance exercise that can help you strengthen your core and stabilizer muscles, and improve your balance and coordination, and prevent falls and injuries. It can also improve your flexibility and range of motion, and reduce your pain and inflammation. Tai chi is a gentle and graceful movement practice that involves shifting your weight and moving your limbs in a coordinated and harmonious way. You can learn tai chi from a qualified instructor, a video, or a book, and practice it in a group or alone, indoors or outdoors. You can start with easy and simple tai chi movements, and gradually increase them as you get more confident and balanced. You can also vary your tai chi exercises, such as different forms, styles, or speeds, to challenge yourself and avoid boredom. You should aim for at least three sessions of tai chi exercises per week, preferably in a safe and supervised environment, doing 10 to 30 minutes

of each session, and repeating 2 to 4 times. You should use proper form and technique, and avoid holding your breath or tensing your muscles.

These are some of the examples and routines of balance exercises for arthritis, but they are not the only ones. You can also try other forms of balance exercises, such as standing on a balance board, a bosu ball, or a wobble cushion, or using a stability ball, a medicine ball, or a kettlebell, as long as they are suitable and safe for you.

The ways to track and measure your progress and results

To make the most of your exercise and physical therapy program, you should track and measure your progress and results regularly and objectively. This can help you evaluate the effectiveness and safety of your exercise and physical therapy, and adjust them accordingly. It can also motivate you to continue and improve your exercise and physical therapy, and celebrate your achievements and milestones.

There are different ways to track and measure your progress and results, such as:

1. **Keeping a journal or a log**: You can record your exercise and physical therapy sessions, such as the type, frequency, intensity, and duration of your exercise and physical therapy, and how you felt during and after them. You can also note any changes or problems with your exercise and physical therapy, and any feedback or suggestions from your doctor or physical therapist. You can review your journal or log periodically, and look for patterns, trends, or areas of improvement.

2. **Using a tracker or a device**: You can use a tracker or a device, such as a pedometer, a heart rate monitor, a fitness watch, or a smartphone app, to measure and monitor your exercise and physical therapy parameters, such as your steps, distance, speed, calories, heart rate, or blood pressure. You can also use a tracker or a device to set and track your exercise and physical therapy goals, such as your target weight, endurance, or strength. You can compare your tracker or device data with your

baseline and expected values, and see how you are progressing and performing.

3. **Taking a test or a measurement**: You can take a test or a measurement, such as a blood test, a joint aspiration, an x-ray, an ultrasound, an MRI, or a joint function and mobility assessment, to evaluate the condition and status of your joints and muscles, and the impact of your exercise and physical therapy on them. You can also take a test or a measurement, such as a pain scale, a quality of life questionnaire, a depression scale, or a satisfaction survey, to assess the effect of your exercise and physical therapy on your symptoms and well-being. You can compare your test or measurement results with your baseline and expected values, and see how you are improving and benefiting.

These are some of the ways to track and measure your progress and results, but they are not the only ones. You can also use other methods or tools that are appropriate and convenient for you, such as photos, videos, charts, graphs, or badges, to track and measure your progress and results.

You should track and measure your progress and results at least once a month, or more often if needed or recommended by your doctor or physical therapist. You should also share your progress and results with your doctor or physical therapist, and discuss any questions or concerns with them. They can help you interpret and analyze your progress and results, and provide you with feedback and guidance.

In conclusion, exercise and physical therapy are vital parts of arthritis treatment and management. They can help you strengthen your joints and muscles, reduce your pain and inflammation, improve your function and mobility, and enhance your quality of life. Exercise and physical therapy can also help you prevent or delay the progression of arthritis, and reduce the need for medications or surgery.

You learned about the benefits of exercise and physical therapy for arthritis, the best types and frequency of exercise for arthritis, the tips and precautions for exercising safely and avoiding injury, the examples and routines of arthritis-friendly exercises and activities, and the ways to track and measure your progress and results. By exercising and moving more, you can not only improve your physical health, but also your mental and emotional well-being. Exercise and physical therapy can also help you live a more active and fulfilling life, despite your arthritis.

Chapter 4: Stretching and Improving Your Flexibility for Arthritis

If you have arthritis, you may think that stretching is not for you. You may worry that it will cause more pain, inflammation, or damage to your joints. You may also think that you are too stiff, too old, or too limited to benefit from stretching. However, these are all myths that can prevent you from enjoying the many benefits of stretching and improving your flexibility for arthritis. In this chapter, we will explain why stretching is one of the best things you can do for your arthritis, and how it can help you improve your range of motion, prevent contractures, reduce pain, and enhance your quality of life. We will also share with you the best types and frequency of stretching for arthritis, as well as some tips and precautions for stretching safely and effectively. Finally, we will show you some examples and routines of arthritis-friendly stretches and poses that you can do at home, at work, or anywhere you like. By the end of this chapter, you will have a better understanding of how stretching and flexibility can help you manage your arthritis and improve your mobility.

The Benefits of Stretching and Flexibility for Arthritis

Stretching and flexibility are often overlooked aspects of physical activity, especially for people with arthritis. However, they are essential for maintaining and improving your joint health and function. Here are some of the benefits of stretching and flexibility for arthritis:

- **Improving your range of motion**: Range of motion is the degree to which you can move your joints in different directions. Arthritis can cause your joints to become stiff, swollen, and inflamed, limiting your range of motion and making it harder to perform everyday tasks. Stretching can help you loosen up your joints and muscles, increase your blood flow and lubrication, and restore your normal range of motion. This can make it easier for you to move, bend, reach, twist, and turn without pain or difficulty.

- **Preventing contractures**: Contractures are permanent shortening or tightening of your muscles, tendons, or ligaments around your joints, resulting from prolonged immobility, inflammation, or scar tissue. Contractures can cause your joints to become fixed in a bent or straight position, reducing your mobility and function. Stretching can help you prevent contractures by keeping your muscles, tendons, and ligaments flexible and elastic, and preventing them from shrinking or sticking together. This can help you preserve your joint mobility and function, and prevent deformities or disabilities.

- **Reducing pain**: Pain is one of the most common and debilitating symptoms of arthritis. It can interfere with your daily activities, sleep, mood, and overall well-being. Stretching can help you reduce pain by relaxing your muscles, releasing tension, improving your circulation, and stimulating the production of natural painkillers called endorphins. Stretching can also help you cope with pain by distracting you from negative thoughts and emotions, and giving you a sense of control and accomplishment.

- **Enhancing your quality of life**: Stretching and flexibility can have a positive impact on your quality of life, both physically and mentally. Physically, stretching can help you improve your posture, balance, coordination, and stability, which can reduce your risk of falls and injuries. Stretching can also help you improve your fitness, endurance, and strength, which can enable you to participate in more activities and hobbies that you enjoy. Mentally, stretching can help you improve your mood, confidence, and self-esteem, which can reduce your stress, anxiety, and depression. Stretching can also help you improve your cognitive function, memory, and concentration, which can enhance your productivity and performance.

As you can see, stretching and flexibility can offer you many benefits for your arthritis, and can complement other treatments and therapies that you may be using. However, not all stretches are created equal, and some may be more suitable for your arthritis than others.

The Best Types and Frequency of Stretching for Arthritis

There are many types of stretching exercises that you can do for your arthritis, but not all of them are equally effective or appropriate for your condition. Some of the most common types of stretching are:

- **Static stretching**: This is the most common and familiar type of stretching, where you hold a stretch for a certain amount of time, usually 10 to 30 seconds. Static stretching can help you improve your flexibility and range of motion, as well as relax your muscles and reduce tension. However, static stretching can also cause micro-tears in your muscles and tendons, which can increase inflammation and pain. Therefore, static stretching is best done after a warm-up or at the end of your exercise session, when your muscles are warm and pliable. Static stretching is also not recommended for joints that are very inflamed, swollen, or unstable, as it can aggravate your symptoms or cause injury.

- **Dynamic stretching**: This is a type of stretching where you move your joints and muscles through their full range of motion, without holding the stretch. Dynamic stretching can help you improve your mobility, coordination, and blood flow, as well as prepare your muscles and joints for activity. Dynamic stretching is best done before your exercise session, as part of your warm-up, to prevent stiffness and injury. Dynamic stretching is also more suitable for joints that are inflamed, swollen, or unstable, as it does not put too much stress or pressure on them. However, dynamic stretching can also be challenging and risky, especially if you have poor balance, strength, or flexibility. Therefore, dynamic stretching should be done carefully and gradually, with proper guidance and support.

- **Ballistic stretching**: This is a type of stretching where you bounce or jerk your joints and muscles beyond their normal range of motion, using momentum and force. Ballistic stretching can help you increase your power, speed, and agility, as well as improve your flexibility and range of motion. However, ballistic stretching can also be very dangerous and harmful, especially for people with arthritis, as it can cause damage to your joints, muscles, tendons, and ligaments, and increase your risk of injury, inflammation, and pain. Therefore, ballistic stretching is not recommended for arthritis, and should be avoided at all costs.

- **Proprioceptive neuromuscular facilitation (PNF) stretching**: This is a type of stretching where you contract and relax your muscles in a specific sequence, while applying resistance or pressure to the stretch. PNF stretching can help you improve your flexibility, range of motion, and muscle strength, as well as reduce muscle spasms and pain. PNF stretching is best done with a partner, such as a physical therapist, who can assist you with the technique and provide feedback. PNF stretching can also be done with a strap, band, or towel, if you do not have a partner. However, PNF stretching can also be complex and intense, and may not be suitable for everyone. Therefore, PNF stretching should be done with caution and supervision, and only after you have mastered the basic stretches.

As you can see, there are pros and cons to each type of stretching, and you need to choose the ones that are best for your arthritis, goals, and preferences. You also need to consider the frequency of your stretching, which depends on several factors, such as your current level of flexibility, the severity of your arthritis, and the type of exercise you are doing. In general, the following guidelines can help you determine how often you should stretch:

- **Stretch at least three times a week**: This is the minimum frequency that you need to maintain and improve your flexibility and range of motion, and prevent contractures. You can stretch more often if you want to, as long as you do not overdo it or cause pain or injury.

- **Stretch before and after your exercise session**: This can help you prepare your muscles and joints for activity, and prevent stiffness and soreness after exercise. However, you need to adjust the type and duration of your stretching according to the phase of your exercise session. Before exercise, do dynamic stretching for 5 to 10 minutes, as part of your warm-up. After exercise, do static stretching for 10 to 15 minutes, as part of your cool-down.

- **Stretch on your rest days**: This can help you recover from your exercise session, and maintain your flexibility and range of motion. On your rest days, you can do static or PNF stretching for 15 to 20 minutes, or as long as you feel comfortable. You can also do some gentle dynamic stretching, such as yoga or tai chi, if you prefer.

By following these guidelines, you can optimize the benefits of stretching and flexibility for your arthritis, and avoid the potential risks and pitfalls. However, you also need to be aware of some tips and precautions for stretching safely and effectively.

Tips and Precautions for Stretching Safely and Effectively

Stretching can be a great way to improve your flexibility and mobility for arthritis, but only if you do it correctly and safely. Otherwise, you may end up hurting yourself or worsening your condition. Here are some tips and precautions that you should follow when stretching for arthritis:

- **Consult your doctor or physical therapist**: Before you start any stretching program, you should consult your doctor or physical therapist, who can assess your joint health and function, and recommend the best types and frequency of stretching for you. They can also teach you the proper technique and form, and monitor your progress and response. They can also advise you on when to stop or modify your stretching, depending on your symptoms and flare-ups.

- **Listen to your body**: Stretching should feel good, not bad. You should feel a gentle pull or tension in your muscles, not pain or discomfort in your joints. If you feel any pain, stop or ease off the stretch immediately. Do not force or overstretch your joints, as this can cause damage or injury. You should also avoid stretching when your joints are very inflamed, swollen, or hot, as this can aggravate your condition. Wait until your inflammation subsides, or use ice or medication to reduce it, before stretching.

- **Warm up before stretching**: Stretching cold muscles and joints can increase your risk of injury and pain. Therefore, you should always warm up before stretching, by doing some light aerobic activity, such as walking, cycling, or swimming, for 5 to 10 minutes. This can help you increase your blood flow, lubrication, and temperature, and prepare your muscles and joints for stretching. You can also use heat, such as a hot shower, bath, or pack, to warm up your muscles and joints, but only if they are not inflamed or swollen.

- **Cool down after stretching**: Stretching can cause your muscles and joints to relax and lengthen, which can make them more vulnerable to injury and pain. Therefore, you should always cool down after stretching, by doing some gentle movements, such as rotating your joints, or shaking your limbs, for a few minutes. This can help you restore your normal muscle tone and joint stability, and prevent stiffness and soreness. You can also use cold, such as an ice pack or gel, to cool down your muscles and joints, but only if they are inflamed or swollen.

- **Breathe normally**: Stretching can affect your breathing, as you may tend to hold your breath or breathe shallowly when you stretch. However, this can reduce your oxygen supply, and increase your tension and stress. Therefore, you should breathe normally when you stretch, by inhaling and exhaling deeply and slowly, through your nose or mouth. This can help you relax your muscles and joints, and enhance your stretching experience. You can also use some breathing techniques, such as counting or humming, to regulate your breathing and focus your attention.

- **Be consistent and progressive**: Stretching can only benefit you if you do it regularly and gradually. Therefore, you should be consistent and progressive with your stretching program, by following the frequency and duration that your doctor or physical therapist recommended, and sticking to your schedule. You should also increase the intensity and complexity of your stretching, as you become more flexible and comfortable, by holding the stretch longer, moving the joint further, or adding some resistance or challenge. However, you should always do this slowly and carefully, and avoid making any sudden or drastic changes.

By following these tips and precautions, you can stretch safely and effectively for your arthritis, and maximize the benefits and minimize the risks. However, you also need to know some examples and routines of arthritis-friendly stretches and poses that you can do.

Examples and Routines of Arthritis-Friendly Stretches and Poses

Now that you know the benefits, types, frequency, tips, and precautions of stretching for arthritis, you may be wondering what are some examples and routines of arthritis-friendly stretches and poses that you can do. In this section, we will show you some of the most common and effective stretches and poses for different parts of your body, such as your neck, shoulders, back, hips, knees, and ankles. We will also provide you with some sample routines that you can follow, or modify according to your needs and preferences.

Before you start any of these stretches and poses, make sure that you have warmed up properly, and that you have a comfortable and spacious place to do them. You may also need some props, such as a chair, a wall, a mat, a strap, a band, a towel, a pillow, or a block, to assist you with some of the stretches and poses. You can also use music, aromatherapy, or meditation to enhance your stretching experience.

Neck Stretches and Poses

The neck is one of the most common areas where people with arthritis experience stiffness and pain. Stretching your neck can help you relieve tension, improve your posture, and prevent headaches. Here are some of the most common and effective neck stretches and poses that you can do:

- **Neck rotation**: This is a simple and gentle stretch that can help you improve your neck mobility and flexibility. To do this stretch, sit or stand with your back straight and your shoulders relaxed. Slowly turn your head to the right, as far as you can, without straining your neck. Hold the stretch for 10 to 15 seconds, then slowly return to the center. Repeat on the left side. Do this stretch 3 to 5 times on each side.

- **Neck tilt**: This is another simple and gentle stretch that can help you stretch the sides of your neck and your upper back. To do this stretch, sit or stand with your back straight and your shoulders relaxed. Slowly tilt your head to the right, bringing your right ear toward your right shoulder, as far as you can, without lifting your shoulder or straining your neck. Hold the stretch for 10 to 15 seconds, then slowly return to the center. Repeat on the left side. Do this stretch 3 to 5 times on each side.

- **Neck flexion and extension**: This is a stretch that can help you stretch the front and back of your neck and your chest. To do this stretch, sit or stand with your back straight and your shoulders relaxed. Slowly lower your chin toward your chest, as far as you can, without rounding your back or straining your neck. Hold the stretch for 10 to 15 seconds, then slowly lift your head and look up, as far as you can, without arching your back or straining your neck. Hold the stretch for 10 to 15 seconds, then slowly return to the center. Do this stretch 3 to 5 times.

- **Neck retraction**: This is a stretch that can help you correct your posture and prevent forward head syndrome, which is a common problem for people who spend a lot of time looking at screens or reading. To do this stretch, sit or stand with your back straight and your shoulders relaxed. Slowly pull your head back, as if you are trying to make a double chin, without tilting your head up or down. Hold the stretch for 10 to 15 seconds, then slowly release. Do this stretch 3 to 5 times.

- **Ear to shoulder pose**: This is a yoga pose that can help you stretch the sides of your neck and your upper back, as well as relax your mind and body. To do this pose, sit on the floor or on a mat, with your legs crossed or extended in front of you. Place your right hand on the floor next to your right hip, and your left hand on the top of your head. Slowly tilt your head to the right, bringing your right ear toward your right shoulder, as far as you can, without lifting your shoulder or straining your neck. Gently press your left hand on your head, to deepen the stretch. Hold the pose for 10 to 15 seconds, then slowly release. Repeat on the left side. Do this pose 3 to 5 times on each side.

Shoulder Stretches and Poses

The shoulders are another common area where people with arthritis experience stiffness and pain. Stretching your shoulders can help you improve your upper body mobility and function, and prevent frozen shoulder syndrome. Here are some of the most common and effective shoulder stretches and poses that you can do:

- **Shoulder rolls**: This is a simple and gentle stretch that can help you loosen up your shoulder joints and muscles, and improve your blood flow and lubrication. To do this stretch, sit or stand with your back straight and your shoulders relaxed. Slowly roll your shoulders forward, up, back, and down, in a circular motion, as if you are shrugging. Do this stretch 10 to 15 times, then reverse the direction. Do this stretch 3 to 5 times in each direction.

- **Shoulder stretch**: This is a stretch that can help you stretch the back of your shoulders and your upper arms. To do this stretch, sit or stand with your back straight and your shoulders relaxed. Bring your right arm across your chest, and use your left hand to gently pull your right elbow toward your chest, as far as you can, without twisting your torso or straining your shoulder. Hold the stretch for 10 to 15 seconds, then slowly release. Repeat on the left side. Do this stretch 3 to 5 times on each side.

- **Shoulder rotation**: This is a stretch that can help you stretch the front of your shoulders and your chest. To do this stretch, sit or stand with your back straight and your shoulders relaxed. Clasp your hands behind your back, and lift your arms as high as you can, without arching your back or straining your shoulders. Hold the stretch for 10 to 15 seconds, then slowly lower your arms. Do this stretch 3 to 5 times.

- **Shoulder blade squeeze**: This is a stretch that can help you strengthen your upper back and improve your posture. To do this stretch, sit or stand with your back straight and your shoulders relaxed. Squeeze your shoulder blades together, as if you are trying to hold a pencil between them, without raising your shoulders or sticking your chest out. Hold the stretch for 10 to 15 seconds, then slowly release. Do this stretch 3 to 5 times.

- **Cow face pose**: This is a yoga pose that can help you stretch the sides of your shoulders and your upper arms, as well as improve your shoulder mobility and flexibility. To do this pose, sit on the floor or on a mat, with your legs crossed or extended in front of you. Reach your right arm up, and bend your elbow behind your head, as if you are scratching your back. Reach your left arm down, and bend your elbow behind your back, as if you are reaching for your right hand. Try to clasp your fingers together, or use a strap, band, or towel to bridge the gap. Hold the pose for 10 to 15 seconds, then slowly release. Repeat on the other side. Do this pose 3 to 5 times on each side.

Back Stretches and Poses

The back is another common area where people with arthritis experience stiffness and pain. Stretching your back can help you improve your spine health and function, and prevent lower back pain. Here are some of the most common and effective back stretches and poses that you can do:

- **Back arch**: This is a simple and gentle stretch that can help you stretch the front of your spine and your abdomen. To do this stretch, lie on your back on the floor or on a mat, with your knees bent and your feet flat. Place your hands behind your head, and lift your head and shoulders off the floor, as far as you can, without straining your neck or back. Hold the stretch for 10 to 15 seconds, then slowly lower your head and shoulders. Do this stretch 3 to 5 times.

- **Back twist**: This is a stretch that can help you stretch the sides of your spine and your lower back.

To do this stretch, lie on your back on the floor or on a mat, with your knees bent and your feet flat. Extend your arms to the sides, at shoulder level, palms down. Slowly drop your knees to the right, as far as you can, without lifting your left shoulder or hip. Hold the stretch for 10 to 15 seconds, then slowly bring your knees back to the center. Repeat on the left side. Do this stretch 3 to 5 times on each side.

- **Back extension**: This is a stretch that can help you stretch the back of your spine and your lower back. To do this stretch, lie on your stomach on the floor or on a mat, with your legs straight and your feet together. Place your hands under your shoulders, and push yourself up, as far as you can, without lifting your hips or legs. Hold the stretch for 10 to 15 seconds, then slowly lower yourself down. Do this stretch 3 to 5 times.

- **Back flexion**: This is a stretch that can help you stretch the front of your spine and your chest. To do this stretch, sit on the floor or on a mat, with your legs extended in front of you. Bend your knees and bring your feet close to your buttocks. Wrap your arms around your knees, and hug them to your chest. Slowly lower your head and round your back, as far as you can, without straining your neck or back. Hold the stretch for 10 to 15 seconds, then slowly lift your head and straighten your back. Do this stretch 3 to 5 times.

- **Child's pose**: This is a yoga pose that can help you relax your spine and your lower back, as well as calm your mind and body. To do this pose, kneel on the floor or on a mat, with your knees slightly apart and your feet together. Sit back on your heels, and lean forward, resting your forehead on the floor or on a pillow. Extend your arms in front of you, palms down, or place them by your sides, palms up. Hold the pose for 10 to 15 seconds, or as long as you feel comfortable. Do this pose 3 to 5 times.

<u>**Hip Stretches and Poses**</u>

The hips are another common area where people with arthritis experience stiffness and pain. Stretching your hips can help you improve your lower body mobility and function, and prevent hip osteoarthritis. Here are some of the most common and effective hip stretches and poses that you can do:

- **Hip flexor stretch**: This is a stretch that can help you stretch the front of your hips and your thighs. To do this stretch, kneel on the floor or on a mat, with your right knee bent and your left leg extended behind you. Place your hands on your right thigh, and lean forward, as far as you can, without arching your back or straining your hips. Hold the stretch for 10 to 15 seconds, then slowly return to the starting position. Repeat on the other side. Do this stretch 3 to 5 times on each side.

- **Hip rotator stretch**: This is a stretch that can help you stretch the back of your hips and your buttocks. To do this stretch, sit on the floor or on a mat, with your legs extended in front of you. Bend your right knee and cross your right ankle over your left thigh, just above your knee. Place your right hand on the floor behind you, and your left hand on your right knee. Gently press your right knee down, and twist your torso to the right, as far as you can, without lifting your hips or straining your back. Hold the stretch for 10 to 15 seconds, then slowly return to the center. Repeat on the other side. Do this stretch 3 to 5 times on each side.

- **Hip adductor stretch**: This is a stretch that can help you stretch the inside of your hips and your groin. To do this stretch, sit on the floor or on a mat, with your legs wide apart. Place your hands on the floor in front of you, and lean forward, as far as you can, without rounding your back or straining your hips. Hold the stretch for 10 to 15 seconds, then slowly return to the starting position. Do this stretch 3 to 5 times.

- **Hip abductor stretch**: This is a stretch that can help you stretch the outside of your hips and your thighs. To do this stretch, lie on your back on the floor or on a mat, with your legs straight and your feet together. Bend your right knee and bring it across your body, toward your left shoulder, as far as you can, without lifting your right shoulder or hip. Use your left hand to gently pull your right knee closer to your chest, and your right hand to press your right hip down. Hold the stretch for 10 to 15 seconds, then slowly release. Repeat on the other side. Do this stretch 3 to 5 times on each side.

- **Pigeon pose**: This is a yoga pose that can help you stretch the front and back of your hips and your lower back, as well as improve your hip mobility and flexibility. To do this pose, start on your hands and knees on the floor or on a mat. Slide your right knee forward, between your hands, and bring your right foot toward your left hip. Extend your left leg behind you, and point your toes. Lower your hips to the floor, and adjust your position until you feel a comfortable stretch. You can stay upright, or lean forward and rest your forehead on the floor or on a pillow. Hold the pose for 10 to 15 seconds, or as long as you feel comfortable. Slowly return to the starting position, and switch sides. Do this pose 3 to 5 times on each side.

Knee Stretches and Poses

The knees are another common area where people with arthritis experience stiffness and pain. Stretching your knees can help you improve your lower body mobility and function, and prevent knee osteoarthritis. Here are some of the most common and effective knee stretches and poses that you can do:

- **Knee flexion and extension**: This is a simple and gentle stretch that can help you stretch the front and back of your knees and your thighs. To do this stretch, sit on a chair, with your back straight and your feet flat on the floor. Slowly extend your right leg in front of you, and flex your foot, as far as you can, without locking your knee or straining your leg. Hold the stretch for 10 to 15 seconds, then slowly bend your knee and lower your foot. Repeat on the left side. Do this stretch 3 to 5 times on each side.

- **Knee rotation**: This is a stretch that can help you stretch the sides of your knees and your lower legs. To do this stretch, sit on a chair, with your back straight and your feet flat on the floor. Cross your right ankle over your left knee, and place your right hand on your right knee. Gently press your right knee down, and rotate your right foot in a circular motion, as if you are drawing a circle with your toes. Do this stretch 10 to 15 times, then reverse the direction. Repeat on the other side. Do this stretch 3 to 5 times on each side.

- **Knee hug**: This is a stretch that can help you stretch the back of your knees and your hamstrings. To do this stretch, lie on your back on the floor or on a mat, with your legs straight and your feet together. Bend your right knee and bring it toward your chest, as far as you can, without lifting your left leg or hip. Wrap your arms around your knee, and hug it to your chest. Hold the stretch for 10 to 15 seconds, then slowly lower your leg. Repeat on the other side. Do this stretch 3 to 5 times on each side.

- **Knee to chest pose**: This is a yoga pose that can help you relax your knees and your lower back, as well as calm your mind and body. To do this pose, lie on your back on the floor or on a mat, with your legs straight and your feet together. Bend both knees and bring them toward your chest, as far as you can, without lifting your head or shoulders. Wrap your arms around your knees, and hug them to your chest. Hold the pose for 10 to 15 seconds, or as long as you feel comfortable. Do this pose 3 to 5 times.

Ankle Stretches and Poses

The ankles are another common area where people with arthritis experience stiffness and pain. Stretching your ankles can help you improve your lower body mobility and function, and prevent ankle osteoarthritis. Here are some of the most common and effective ankle stretches and poses that you can do:

- **Ankle flexion and extension**: This is a simple and gentle stretch that can help you stretch the front and back of your ankles and your calves. To do this stretch, sit on a chair, with your back straight and your feet flat on the floor. Slowly lift your right foot off the floor, and flex your ankle, bringing your toes toward your shin, as far as you can, without straining your ankle or leg. Hold the stretch for 10 to 15 seconds, then slowly point your toes, extending your ankle, as far as you can, without straining your ankle or leg. Hold the stretch for 10 to 15 seconds, then slowly lower your foot. Repeat on the left side. Do this stretch 3 to 5 times on each side.

- **Ankle rotation**: This is a stretch that can help you stretch the sides of your ankles and your lower legs. To do this stretch, sit on a chair, with your back straight and your feet flat on the floor. Cross your right ankle over your left knee, and place your right hand on your right ankle. Gently rotate your ankle in a circular motion, as if you are drawing a circle with your toes. Do this stretch 10 to 15 times, then reverse the direction. Repeat on the other side. Do this stretch 3 to 5 times on each side.

- **Ankle inversion and eversion**: This is a stretch that can help you stretch the inside and outside of your ankles and your feet. To do this stretch, sit on a chair, with your back straight and your feet flat on the floor. Cross your right ankle over your left knee, and place your right hand on your right foot. Gently turn your foot inward, as if you are trying to touch your sole to your shin, as far as you can, without straining your ankle or foot. Hold the stretch for 10 to 15 seconds, then gently turn your foot outward, as if you are trying to touch your sole to the floor, as far as you can, without straining your ankle or foot. Hold the stretch for 10 to 15 seconds, then slowly return to the center. Repeat on the other side. Do this stretch 3 to 5 times on each side.

- **Ankle stretch**: This is a stretch that can help you stretch the back of your ankles and your Achilles tendons. To do this stretch, stand facing a wall, with your feet shoulder-width apart. Place your hands on the wall, and step your right foot back, keeping your right leg straight and your right heel on the floor. Bend your left knee and lean forward, until you feel a comfortable stretch in your right calf and ankle. Hold the stretch for 10 to 15 seconds, then slowly return to the starting position. Repeat on the other side. Do this stretch 3 to 5 times on each side.

- **Downward facing dog pose**: This is a yoga pose that can help you stretch the front and back of your ankles and your calves, as well as your spine and your hamstrings. To do this pose, start on your hands and knees on the floor or on a mat, with your hands slightly ahead of your shoulders and your knees slightly behind your hips. Curl your toes under, and lift your hips up, straightening your legs and arms, and forming an inverted V shape with your body. Press your heels down, and lengthen your spine, as far as you can, without locking your knees or elbows. Hold the pose for 10 to 15 seconds, or as long as you feel comfortable. Do this pose 3 to 5 times.

The Ways to Incorporate Stretching into Your Daily Life and Routine

Stretching can be a great way to improve your flexibility and mobility for arthritis, but only if you do it regularly and consistently. However, you may find it hard to fit stretching into your busy and hectic schedule, or you may forget to do it altogether. In this section, we will share with you some ways to incorporate stretching into your daily life and routine, and make it a habit that you can stick to.

- **Set a reminder**: One of the easiest ways to incorporate stretching into your daily life and routine is to set a reminder for yourself, such as an alarm, a notification, a calendar event, or a note. You can set a reminder for a specific time of the day, such as in the morning, before bed, or during your lunch break, or for a specific activity, such as before or after exercise, work, or driving. You can also use a reminder app, such as Copilot, that can help you schedule and track your stretching sessions, and provide you with feedback and encouragement.

- **Make it fun**: Another way to incorporate stretching into your daily life and routine is to make it fun and enjoyable, rather than boring and tedious. You can make it fun by adding some variety, creativity, and challenge to your stretching program, such as trying new stretches and poses, changing the location and environment, using props and music, or joining a class or a group. You can also make it fun by rewarding yourself for your progress and achievements, such as treating yourself to a massage, a movie, or a snack, or sharing your results with your friends or family.

- **Make it convenient**: Another way to incorporate stretching into your daily life and routine is to make it convenient and accessible, rather than inconvenient and difficult. You can make it convenient by choosing stretches and poses that you can do anywhere, anytime, and with minimal equipment, such as in your bed, on your couch, at your desk, or in your car. You can also make it convenient by having some props and tools handy, such as a chair, a wall, a mat, a strap, a band, a towel, a pillow, or a block, that you can use to assist you with your stretching.

- **Make it a priority**: Another way to incorporate stretching into your daily life and routine is to make it a priority and a commitment, rather than an option and an excuse. You can make it a priority by setting a goal and a plan for your stretching program, such as how often, how long, and how intense you want to stretch, and what benefits and outcomes you want to achieve. You can also make it a priority by finding a partner, a coach, or a mentor, who can support you, motivate you, and hold you accountable for your stretching.

By following these ways, you can incorporate stretching into your daily life and routine, and make it a habit that you can stick to. Stretching can help you improve your flexibility and mobility for arthritis, and enhance your quality of life, both physically and mentally.

Chapter 5: Using Complementary and Alternative Therapies for Arthritis

Arthritis is a chronic condition that affects millions of people worldwide. It causes inflammation, pain, stiffness, and reduced mobility in the joints. While there is no cure for arthritis, there are many ways to manage its symptoms and improve your quality of life. One of the ways to cope with arthritis is to use complementary and alternative therapies. These are methods of healing that are not part of conventional medicine, but can be used alongside it to enhance your well-being. Complementary and alternative therapies can offer various benefits for people with arthritis, such as:

- Reducing pain and inflammation.
- Improving joint function and flexibility.
- Relieving stress and anxiety.
- Boosting mood and energy.
- Supporting overall health and immunity

In this chapter, we will explore the definition and scope of complementary and alternative therapies for arthritis, the evidence and research behind each therapy and how they work, the most popular and effective therapies for arthritis, such as acupuncture, massage, yoga, meditation, and aromatherapy, the tips and precautions for choosing and using each therapy safely and appropriately, and the ways to combine and integrate different therapies for optimal results.

What are Complementary and Alternative Therapies?

Complementary and alternative therapies (CATs) are a broad range of practices, products, and systems that are not considered part of mainstream medicine, but can be used to complement or replace it. According to the National Center for Complementary and Integrative Health (NCCIH), CATs can be classified into two categories:

- **Natural products**: These are substances that come from plants, animals, or minerals, such as herbs, vitamins, minerals, probiotics, and dietary supplements.

- **Mind and body practices**: These are techniques that involve the interaction of the mind, body, and environment, such as acupuncture, massage, yoga, meditation, tai chi, qi gong, biofeedback, hypnosis, and guided imagery.

Some CATs are based on ancient traditions or cultures, such as traditional Chinese medicine, Ayurveda, or Native American healing. Others are based on modern theories or innovations, such as homeopathy, naturopathy, or energy medicine. The use of CATs is very common among people with arthritis. According to a survey by the Arthritis Foundation, more than half of the respondents reported using at least one type of CAT in the past year, and more than 80% said they were interested in learning more about them. The most commonly used CATs were natural products, massage, meditation, and yoga.

How Do Complementary and Alternative Therapies Work?

The mechanisms of action of CATs are not fully understood by science, and may vary depending on the type and quality of the therapy, the individual characteristics of the user, and the context of the use. However, some possible explanations for how CATs work are:

- **Modulating the nervous system**: Some CATs, such as acupuncture, massage, and meditation, may work by stimulating or relaxing the nerves that control pain, inflammation, and muscle tension. They may also affect the levels of neurotransmitters, such as endorphins, serotonin, and dopamine, that regulate mood, stress, and sleep.

- **Enhancing the immune system**: Some CATs, such as natural products, yoga, and tai chi, may work by boosting the body's natural defenses against infections, inflammation, and oxidative stress. They may also modulate the activity of immune cells, such as T cells, B cells, and natural killer cells, that are involved in autoimmune diseases like rheumatoid arthritis.

- **Improving the biomechanics**: Some CATs, such as massage, yoga, and tai chi, may work by improving the alignment, posture, and movement of the joints, muscles, and tendons. They may also increase the blood flow, oxygen, and nutrients to the affected tissues, and facilitate the removal of waste products and toxins.

- **Changing the perception of pain**: Some CATs, such as meditation, hypnosis, and guided imagery, may work by altering the way the brain processes and responds to pain signals. They may also enhance the coping skills, self-efficacy, and resilience of the user, and reduce the negative emotions, such as fear, anger, and depression, that can amplify pain.

- **Influencing the energy fields**: Some CATs, such as acupuncture, qi gong, and energy medicine, may work by affecting the subtle energies that flow through and around the body, according to some traditions and beliefs. They may also balance the yin and yang, or the positive and negative forces, that govern the health and harmony of the body, mind, and spirit.

The Most Popular and Effective Therapies for Arthritis

There are many types of CATs that can be used for arthritis, but some are more popular and effective than others. Here are some of the most widely used and researched CATs for arthritis, and their benefits and drawbacks:

- **Acupuncture**: This is a technique that involves inserting thin needles into specific points on the skin, called acupoints, to stimulate the flow of energy, or qi, in the body. Acupuncture is one of the oldest and most widely used CATs in the world, and is based on the principles of traditional Chinese medicine. Acupuncture can help reduce pain, inflammation, and stiffness in people with arthritis, especially osteoarthritis of the knee, hip, and hand. It can also improve the function and quality of life of the users. The effects of acupuncture may last for several weeks or months after the treatment. Acupuncture is generally safe and well-tolerated, but some risks include bleeding, bruising, infection, and nerve damage. Acupuncture should be performed by a qualified and licensed practitioner, and the needles should be sterile and disposable.

- **Massage**: This is a technique that involves applying pressure, friction, and movement to the soft tissues of the body, such as the muscles, tendons, and ligaments, to relax and heal them. Massage can be done by hand, or by using tools, such as rollers, balls, or devices. Massage can help relieve pain, inflammation, and stiffness in people with arthritis, especially osteoarthritis of the neck, back, shoulder, and knee. It can also improve the circulation, flexibility, and range of motion of the joints, and reduce stress and anxiety. The effects of massage may last for several hours or days after the session. Massage is generally safe and enjoyable, but some risks include soreness, bruising, swelling, and allergic reactions. Massage should be done by a trained and certified therapist, and the pressure and technique should be adjusted to the user's comfort and preference.

- **Yoga**: This is a practice that involves performing physical postures, breathing exercises, and meditation, to harmonize the body, mind, and spirit. Yoga is one of the oldest and most popular CATs in the world, and is based on the philosophy of Hinduism. Yoga can help improve pain, inflammation, and stiffness in people with arthritis, especially rheumatoid arthritis and osteoarthritis of the knee. It can also improve the strength, balance, and flexibility of the joints, and enhance the mood, energy, and well-being of the users. The effects of yoga may last for several weeks or months after the practice. Yoga is generally safe and adaptable, but some risks include injury, strain, and aggravation of existing conditions. Yoga should be done under the guidance of a qualified and experienced instructor, and the style, level, and duration should be suitable for the user's ability and goal.

- **Meditation**: This is a technique that involves focusing the attention on a chosen object, such as the breath, a word, or a sound, to calm the mind and body. Meditation is one of the oldest and most widely practiced CATs in the world, and is based on various religious and spiritual traditions. Meditation can help reduce pain, inflammation, and stiffness in people with arthritis, especially rheumatoid arthritis and osteoarthritis of the knee. It can also improve the psychological and emotional aspects of living with arthritis, such as stress, anxiety, depression, and coping skills. The effects of meditation may last for several hours or days after the session. Meditation is generally safe and easy to learn, but some risks include distraction, boredom, and frustration. Meditation should be done in a quiet and comfortable place, and the type, frequency, and duration should be tailored to the user's preference and goal.

- **Aromatherapy**: This is a technique that involves inhaling or applying natural oils extracted from plants, such as flowers, herbs, or fruits, to enhance the health and well-being of the user. Aromatherapy is one of the oldest and most widely used CATs in the world, and is based on the belief that different scents have different effects on the body and mind. Aromatherapy can help ease pain, inflammation, and stiffness in people with arthritis, especially osteoarthritis of the knee, hip, and hand. It can also improve the mood, sleep, and relaxation of the users. The effects of aromatherapy may last for several minutes or hours after the exposure. Aromatherapy is generally safe and pleasant, but some risks include allergic reactions, skin irritation, and drug interactions. Aromatherapy should be done with high-quality and pure oils, and the dosage and method should be appropriate for the user's condition and sensitivity.

- **Tai chi**: This is a practice that involves performing slow and graceful movements, coordinated with breathing and mental focus, to balance the energy and harmony of the body, mind, and spirit. Tai chi is one of the oldest and most popular CATs in the world, and is based on the principles of traditional Chinese medicine. Tai chi can help improve pain, inflammation, and stiffness in people with arthritis, especially osteoarthritis of the knee, hip, and hand. It can also improve the strength, balance, and flexibility of the joints, and reduce the risk of falls and injuries. The effects of tai chi may last for several weeks or months after the practice. Tai chi is generally safe and adaptable, but some risks include overexertion, strain, and aggravation of existing conditions. Tai chi should be done under the guidance of a qualified and experienced instructor, and the style, level, and duration should be suitable for the user's ability and goal.

- **Biofeedback**: This is a technique that involves using sensors and devices to monitor and display the physiological signals of the body, such as heart rate, blood pressure, muscle tension, skin temperature, and brain waves, to help the user learn to control them voluntarily. Biofeedback is one of the most modern and scientific CATs in the world, and is based on the theory of operant conditioning. Biofeedback can help reduce pain, inflammation, and stiffness in people with arthritis, especially rheumatoid arthritis and osteoarthritis of the knee. It can also improve the relaxation, stress management, and coping skills of the users. The effects of biofeedback may last for several weeks or months after the training. Biofeedback is generally safe and effective, but some risks include equipment malfunction, user frustration, and dependency. Biofeedback should be done with the help of a trained and certified therapist, and the type, frequency, and duration should be customized to the user's condition and goal.

- **Hypnosis**: This is a technique that involves inducing a state of altered consciousness, in which the user becomes more receptive to suggestions, such as positive affirmations, imagery, or commands, to change their behavior, thoughts, or feelings. Hypnosis is one of the oldest and most controversial CATs in the world, and is based on the power of the subconscious mind. Hypnosis can help reduce pain, inflammation, and stiffness in people with arthritis, especially rheumatoid arthritis and osteoarthritis of the knee. It can also improve the psychological and emotional aspects of living with arthritis, such as anxiety, depression, self-esteem, and coping skills. The effects of hypnosis may last for several hours or days after the session. Hypnosis is generally safe and harmless, but some risks include false memories, adverse reactions, and ethical issues. Hypnosis should be done by a qualified and trustworthy practitioner, and the user should be fully informed and consented to the process and the outcome.

- **Guided imagery**: This is a technique that involves using mental images, sounds, or words, to create a positive and realistic scenario, in which the user can achieve their desired goals, such as pain relief, healing, or relaxation. Guided imagery is one of the simplest and most accessible CATs in the world, and is based on the principle of visualization. Guided imagery can help reduce pain, inflammation, and stiffness in people with arthritis, especially rheumatoid arthritis and osteoarthritis of the knee. It can also improve the mood, sleep, and well-being of the users. The effects of guided imagery may last for several hours or days after the session. Guided imagery is generally safe and easy to do, but some risks include distraction, boredom, and unrealistic expectations. Guided imagery can be done by listening to a recorded script, reading a book, or following the instructions of a therapist, and the user should choose a comfortable and quiet place, and a suitable and appealing theme.

- **Probiotics**: These are live microorganisms, such as bacteria or yeast, that can be consumed through foods, such as yogurt, kefir, or kimchi, or supplements, to improve the health and balance of the gut flora. Probiotics are one of the most popular and promising CATs in the world, and are based on the concept of the gut-brain axis. Probiotics can help reduce pain, inflammation, and stiffness in people with arthritis, especially rheumatoid arthritis and psoriatic arthritis. They can also improve the immune system, digestion, and metabolism of the users. The effects of probiotics may last for several weeks or months after the intake. Probiotics are generally safe and well-tolerated, but some risks include bloating, gas, diarrhea, and infection. Probiotics should be taken with caution by people with compromised immune systems, and the type, dose, and quality should be appropriate for the user's condition and goal.

- **Homeopathy**: This is a system of medicine that involves using highly diluted substances, usually derived from plants, animals, or minerals, to stimulate the body's natural healing response. Homeopathy is one of the oldest and most controversial CATs in the world, and is based on the principle of "like cures like". Homeopathy can help reduce pain, inflammation, and stiffness in people with arthritis, especially osteoarthritis of the knee, hip, and hand. It can also improve the mood, sleep, and well-being of the users. The effects of homeopathy may vary depending on the individual and the remedy. Homeopathy is generally safe and harmless, but some risks include lack of scientific evidence, placebo effect, and adverse reactions. Homeopathy should be done by a qualified and registered practitioner, and the remedy, potency, and frequency should be specific to the user's symptoms and constitution.

- **Naturopathy**: This is a system of medicine that involves using natural and holistic methods, such as diet, lifestyle, herbs, supplements, hydrotherapy, and physical therapies, to promote the self-healing ability of the body. Naturopathy is one of the most modern and comprehensive CATs in the world, and is based on the philosophy of vitalism. Naturopathy can help improve pain, inflammation, and stiffness in people with arthritis, especially rheumatoid arthritis and osteoarthritis of the knee, hip, and hand. It can also address the underlying causes and risk factors of arthritis, such as obesity, inflammation, and oxidative stress. The effects of naturopathy may last for several weeks or months after the treatment. Naturopathy is generally safe and effective, but some risks include interaction with conventional drugs, misdiagnosis, and overuse of supplements. Naturopathy should be done by a trained and licensed naturopathic doctor, and the treatment plan should be individualized and monitored for the user's condition and goal.

- **Energy medicine**: This is a technique that involves using various forms of energy, such as electricity, magnetism, light, sound, or vibration, to influence the health and function of the body. Energy medicine is one of the most modern and diverse CATs in the world, and is based on the concept of biofield. Energy medicine can help improve pain, inflammation, and stiffness in people with arthritis, especially rheumatoid arthritis and osteoarthritis of the knee, hip, and hand. It can also stimulate the healing and regeneration of the tissues, and balance the energy flow and harmony of the body, mind, and spirit. The effects of energy medicine may vary depending on the type and intensity of the energy, and the individual response of the user. Energy medicine is generally safe and non-invasive, but some risks include interference with pacemakers, implants, or other devices, skin irritation, and discomfort. Energy medicine should be done by a qualified and experienced practitioner, and the user should be informed and consented to the procedure and the outcome.

- **Ayurveda**: This is a system of medicine that involves using natural and holistic methods, such as diet, lifestyle, herbs, oils, massage, and cleansing, to balance the three doshas, or the fundamental energies, of the body, namely vata, pitta, and kapha. Ayurveda is one of the oldest and most comprehensive CATs in the world, and is based on the philosophy of Hinduism. Ayurveda can help improve pain, inflammation, and stiffness in people with arthritis, especially rheumatoid arthritis and osteoarthritis of the knee, hip, and hand. It can also address the root causes and risk factors of arthritis, such as toxins, stress, and imbalance of the doshas. The effects of Ayurveda may last for several weeks or months after the treatment. Ayurveda is generally safe and effective, but some risks include contamination, adulteration, and interaction with conventional drugs. Ayurveda should be done by a trained and licensed ayurvedic doctor, and the treatment plan should be individualized and monitored for the user's condition and constitution.

- **Traditional Chinese medicine**: This is a system of medicine that involves using natural and holistic methods, such as herbs, acupuncture, moxibustion, cupping, massage, and exercise, to balance the yin and yang, or the opposite and complementary forces, of the body, and to regulate the flow of qi, or the vital energy, in the body. Traditional Chinese medicine is one of the oldest and most comprehensive CATs in the world, and is based on the principles of Taoism. Traditional Chinese medicine can help improve pain, inflammation, and stiffness in people with arthritis, especially rheumatoid arthritis and osteoarthritis of the knee, hip, and hand. It can also address the underlying causes and risk factors of arthritis, such as dampness, cold, heat, and stagnation of qi. The effects of traditional Chinese medicine may last for several weeks or months after the treatment. Traditional Chinese medicine is generally safe and effective, but some risks include toxicity, infection, and interaction with conventional drugs. Traditional Chinese medicine should be done by a qualified and licensed practitioner, and the diagnosis and treatment should be based on the user's symptoms and constitution.

- **Chiropractic**: This is a technique that involves manipulating the spine and other joints of the body, using the hands or special instruments, to correct their alignment and function. Chiropractic is one of the most modern and popular CATs in the world, and is based on the theory of vertebral subluxation.

Chiropractic can help improve pain, inflammation, and stiffness in people with arthritis, especially osteoarthritis of the neck, back, and knee. It can also improve the nerve conduction, blood circulation, and posture of the users. The effects of chiropractic may last for several hours or days after the adjustment. Chiropractic is generally safe and effective, but some risks include soreness, injury, and stroke. Chiropractic should be done by a trained and licensed chiropractor, and the user should inform them of their medical history and condition.

- **Reiki**: This is a technique that involves transferring universal life force energy, or ki, from the practitioner to the user, through the hands or the eyes, to promote healing and well-being. Reiki is one of the most modern and spiritual CATs in the world, and is based on the teachings of Mikao Usui. Reiki can help reduce pain, inflammation, and stiffness in people with arthritis, especially rheumatoid arthritis and osteoarthritis of the knee, hip, and hand. It can also improve the mood, sleep, and relaxation of the users. The effects of Reiki may vary depending on the individual and the session. Reiki is generally safe and non-invasive, but some risks include emotional distress, fatigue, and placebo effect. Reiki should be done by a qualified and attuned practitioner, and the user should be open and receptive to the energy.

- **Music therapy**: This is a technique that involves using music, such as listening, singing, playing, or composing, to improve the physical, mental, and emotional health of the user. Music therapy is one of the most modern and creative CATs in the world, and is based on the power of sound and rhythm. Music therapy can help reduce pain, inflammation, and stiffness in people with arthritis, especially rheumatoid arthritis and osteoarthritis of the knee, hip, and hand. It can also improve the mood, memory, and cognition of the users. The effects of music therapy may last for several minutes or hours after the session. Music therapy is generally safe and enjoyable, but some risks include noise-induced hearing loss, distraction, and annoyance. Music therapy should be done by a trained and certified music therapist, and the user should choose a suitable and appealing genre, style, and tempo.

- **Hydrotherapy**: This is a technique that involves using water, in various forms, temperatures, and pressures, to treat various conditions and improve the health and well-being of the user. Hydrotherapy is one of the oldest and most common CATs in the world, and is based on the principle of thermoregulation. Hydrotherapy can help reduce pain, inflammation, and stiffness in people with arthritis, especially osteoarthritis of the knee, hip, and hand. It can also improve the circulation, relaxation, and detoxification of the users. The effects of hydrotherapy may last for several minutes or hours after the session. Hydrotherapy is generally safe and accessible, but some risks include infection, dehydration, and thermal injury. Hydrotherapy should be done with caution by people with cardiovascular or respiratory problems, and the type, temperature, and duration should be appropriate for the user's condition and tolerance.

- **Herbal medicine**: This is a technique that involves using plants, or parts of plants, such as leaves, flowers, roots, seeds, or bark, to treat various conditions and improve the health and well-being of the user. Herbal medicine is one of the oldest and most widely used CATs in the world, and is based on the knowledge and experience of different cultures and traditions. Herbal medicine can help reduce pain, inflammation, and stiffness in people with arthritis, especially rheumatoid arthritis and osteoarthritis of the knee, hip, and hand. It can also address the underlying causes and risk factors of arthritis, such as infection, inflammation, and oxidative stress. The effects of herbal medicine may vary depending on the individual and the herb. Herbal medicine is generally safe and natural, but some risks include toxicity, allergy, and interaction with conventional drugs. Herbal medicine should be done with the advice of a qualified and knowledgeable practitioner, and the quality, dose, and preparation should be standardized and verified.

- **Dietary supplements**: These are products that contain one or more ingredients, such as vitamins, minerals, amino acids, enzymes, or other substances, that are intended to supplement the diet and provide health benefits to the user. Dietary supplements are one of the most popular and controversial CATs in the world, and are based on the concept of nutritional deficiency or enhancement. Dietary supplements can help reduce pain, inflammation, and stiffness in people with arthritis, especially rheumatoid arthritis and osteoarthritis of the knee, hip, and hand. They can also support the overall health and immunity of the users. The effects of dietary supplements may vary depending on the individual and the supplement. Dietary supplements are generally safe and convenient, but some risks include overdose, side effects, and interaction with conventional drugs. Dietary supplements should be taken with caution by people with medical conditions or allergies, and the type, dose, and quality should be appropriate for the user's condition and goal.

- **Magnets**: These are objects that produce a magnetic field, which can be applied to the body, either directly or indirectly, to improve the health and function of the body. Magnets are one of the most modern and controversial CATs in the world, and are based on the concept of biomagnetism. Magnets can help reduce pain, inflammation, and stiffness in people with arthritis, especially osteoarthritis of the knee, hip, and hand. They can also improve the blood flow, oxygen, and nutrients to the affected tissues, and stimulate the healing and regeneration of the cells. The effects of magnets may vary depending on the type, strength, and duration of the magnet, and the individual response of the user. Magnets are generally safe and easy to use, but some risks include interference with pacemakers, implants, or other devices, skin irritation, and placebo effect. Magnets should be used with caution by people with cardiovascular or neurological problems, and the quality, dose, and placement should be appropriate for the user's condition and goal.

- **Essential oils**: These are concentrated liquids extracted from plants, such as flowers, herbs, or fruits, that have distinctive aromas and properties, and can be used for various purposes, such as healing, beauty, or cleaning. Essential oils are one of the oldest and most widely used CATs in the world, and are based on the concept of aromatherapy. Essential oils can help reduce pain, inflammation, and stiffness in people with arthritis, especially rheumatoid arthritis and osteoarthritis of the knee, hip, and hand. They can also improve the mood, sleep, and relaxation of the users. The effects of essential oils may last for several minutes or hours after the application or inhalation. Essential oils are generally safe and natural, but some risks include allergic reactions, skin irritation, and drug interactions. Essential oils should be used with care by people with sensitive skin or allergies, and the quality, dose, and method should be suitable for the user's condition and preference.

- **Ginger**: This is a spice that comes from the root of a plant, and can be used as a food, a drink, or a supplement, to improve the health and well-being of the user. Ginger is one of the oldest and most common CATs in the world, and is based on the concept of anti-inflammatory. Ginger can help reduce pain, inflammation, and stiffness in people with arthritis, especially rheumatoid arthritis and osteoarthritis of the knee, hip, and hand. It can also improve the digestion, metabolism, and immunity of the users. The effects of ginger may last for several hours or days after the intake. Ginger is generally safe and delicious, but some risks include heartburn, nausea, and bleeding. Ginger should be taken with moderation by people with stomach ulcers or blood disorders, and the quality, dose, and preparation should be appropriate for the user's condition and goal.

- **Turmeric**: This is a spice that comes from the root of a plant, and can be used as a food, a drink, or a supplement, to improve the health and well-being of the user. Turmeric is one of the oldest and most common CATs in the world, and is based on the concept of anti-inflammatory. Turmeric can help reduce pain, inflammation, and stiffness in people with arthritis, especially rheumatoid arthritis and osteoarthritis of the knee, hip, and hand. It can also improve the immune system, digestion, and metabolism of the users. The effects of turmeric may last for several hours or days after the intake. Turmeric is generally safe and delicious, but some risks include stomach upset, bleeding, and interaction with conventional drugs. Turmeric should be taken with caution by people with gallstones or blood disorders, and the quality, dose, and preparation should be appropriate for the user's condition and goal.

- **Glucosamine and chondroitin**: These are substances that are naturally found in the cartilage, the connective tissue that cushions the joints, and can be taken as supplements to improve the health and function of the joints. Glucosamine and chondroitin are some of the most popular and researched CATs in the world, and are based on the concept of joint repair. Glucosamine and chondroitin can help reduce pain, inflammation, and stiffness in people with arthritis, especially osteoarthritis of the knee, hip, and hand. They can also slow down the progression of cartilage degeneration, and improve the mobility and quality of life of the users. The effects of glucosamine and chondroitin may vary depending on the individual and the supplement. Glucosamine and chondroitin are generally safe and well-tolerated, but some risks include allergic reactions, gastrointestinal problems, and interaction with conventional drugs. Glucosamine and chondroitin should be taken with care by people with shellfish allergy or diabetes, and the type, dose, and quality should be appropriate for the user's condition and goal.

- **Omega-3 fatty acids**: These are essential fats that are found in certain foods, such as fish, nuts, seeds, and oils, or supplements, and can provide various health benefits to the user. Omega-3 fatty acids are some of the most popular and promising CATs in the world, and are based on the concept of anti-inflammatory. Omega-3 fatty acids can help reduce pain, inflammation, and stiffness in people with arthritis, especially rheumatoid arthritis and osteoarthritis of the knee, hip, and hand. They can also improve the cardiovascular, cognitive, and emotional health of the users. The effects of omega-3 fatty acids may last for several weeks or months after the intake. Omega-3 fatty acids are generally safe and beneficial, but some risks include fishy taste, burping, and interaction with conventional drugs. Omega-3 fatty acids should be taken with caution by people with bleeding disorders or seafood allergy, and the type, dose, and quality should be appropriate for the user's condition and goal.

- **Green tea**: This is a beverage that is made from the leaves of the Camellia sinensis plant, and can be consumed hot or cold, to improve the health and well-being of the user. Green tea is one of the oldest and most common CATs in the world, and is based on the concept of antioxidant. Green tea can help reduce pain, inflammation, and stiffness in people with arthritis, especially rheumatoid arthritis and osteoarthritis of the knee, hip, and hand. It can also improve the immune system, metabolism, and cognition of the users. The effects of green tea may last for several hours or days after the intake. Green tea is generally safe and delicious, but some risks include caffeine, tannins, and interaction with conventional drugs. Green tea should be taken with moderation by people with insomnia, anxiety, or anemia, and the quality, dose, and preparation should be appropriate for the user's condition and goal.

- **Capsaicin**: This is a substance that is found in chili peppers, and can be used as a food, a cream, or a patch, to improve the health and function of the body. Capsaicin is one of the most modern and spicy CATs in the world, and is based on the concept of counterirritant. Capsaicin can help reduce pain, inflammation, and stiffness in people with arthritis, especially osteoarthritis of the knee, hip, and hand. It can also improve the blood flow, oxygen, and nutrients to the affected tissues, and stimulate the release of endorphins, the natural painkillers of the body. The effects of capsaicin may vary depending on the individual and the product. Capsaicin is generally safe and effective, but some risks include burning, itching, and irritation. Capsaicin should be used with care by people with sensitive skin or eyes, and the quality, dose, and method should be suitable for the user's condition and tolerance.

- **Boswellia**: This is a resin that is obtained from the bark of a tree, and can be used as a food, a drink, or a supplement, to improve the health and well-being of the user. Boswellia is one of the oldest and most sacred CATs in the world, and is based on the concept of anti-inflammatory. Boswellia can help reduce pain, inflammation, and stiffness in people with arthritis, especially rheumatoid arthritis and osteoarthritis of the knee, hip, and hand. It can also improve the immune system, digestion, and mood of the users. The effects of boswellia may last for several hours or days after the intake. Boswellia is generally safe and natural, but some risks include stomach upset, allergy, and interaction with conventional drugs. Boswellia should be taken with caution by people with stomach ulcers or blood disorders, and the quality, dose, and preparation should be appropriate for the user's condition and goal.

- **Apple cider vinegar**: This is a liquid that is made from fermented apple juice, and can be used as a food, a drink, or a topical application, to improve the health and well-being of the user. Apple cider vinegar is one of the oldest and most common CATs in the world, and is based on the concept of acid-base balance. Apple cider vinegar can help reduce pain, inflammation, and stiffness in people with arthritis, especially osteoarthritis of the knee, hip, and hand. It can also improve the digestion, metabolism, and detoxification of the users. The effects of apple cider vinegar may last for several hours or days after the intake or application. Apple cider vinegar is generally safe and inexpensive, but some risks include erosion of tooth enamel, irritation of the throat, and interaction with conventional drugs. Apple cider vinegar should be taken with moderation by people with acid reflux or diabetes, and the quality, dose, and method should be appropriate for the user's condition and goal.

- **Bee venom therapy**: This is a technique that involves injecting or applying the venom of honeybees, either directly or indirectly, to the affected joints or muscles, to improve the health and function of the body. Bee venom therapy is one of the oldest and most exotic CATs in the world, and is based on the concept of immunotherapy. Bee venom therapy can help reduce pain, inflammation, and stiffness in people with arthritis, especially rheumatoid arthritis and osteoarthritis of the knee, hip, and hand. It can also stimulate the immune system, blood circulation, and nerve conduction of the users. The effects of bee venom therapy may vary depending on the individual and the dose. Bee venom therapy is generally safe and effective, but some risks include allergic reactions, infection, and anaphylaxis. Bee venom therapy should be done by a qualified and experienced practitioner, and the user should be tested and monitored for their sensitivity and response.

- **Cannabidiol (CBD)**: This is a substance that is derived from the cannabis plant, and can be used as an oil, a capsule, a cream, or a gummy, to improve the health and well-being of the user. CBD is one of the most modern and popular CATs in the world, and is based on the concept of endocannabinoid system. CBD can help reduce pain, inflammation, and stiffness in people with arthritis, especially rheumatoid arthritis and osteoarthritis of the knee, hip, and hand. It can also improve the mood, sleep, and relaxation of the users. The effects of CBD may last for several hours or days after the intake or application. CBD is generally safe and well-tolerated, but some risks include drowsiness, dry mouth, and interaction with conventional drugs. CBD should be taken with caution by people with liver problems or psychiatric disorders, and the type, dose, and quality should be appropriate for the user's condition and goal.

Tips and Precautions for Choosing and Using Each Therapy Safely and Appropriately

Before starting any complementary and alternative therapy, consult your doctor and inform them of your medical history, condition, and medications. Some therapies may not be suitable or safe for you, or may interact with your conventional treatment. Choose a qualified and reputable practitioner or therapist for your therapy, and check their credentials, experience, and reviews. Ask them about their training, certification, and license, and what to expect from the therapy. Communicate your needs, preferences, and feedback, and follow their instructions and advice.

Choose a high-quality and reliable product or supplement for your therapy, and check its ingredients, dosage, and expiration date. Read the label and the instructions carefully, and follow them strictly. Avoid products or supplements that make unrealistic or exaggerated claims, or that do not have clear or credible information. Start with a low dose or intensity of your therapy, and gradually increase it as you feel comfortable and confident. Do not exceed the recommended dose or duration of your therapy, and stop or reduce it if you experience any adverse effects or discomfort. Monitor your response and progress, and keep a record of your therapy.

Be aware of the potential risks and side effects of your therapy, and report them to your doctor or therapist as soon as possible. Some common signs of a problem include pain, swelling, redness, itching, rash, bleeding, infection, nausea, vomiting, diarrhea, headache, dizziness, fatigue, or mood changes. Seek immediate medical attention if you have a severe or life-threatening reaction, such as difficulty breathing, chest pain, or loss of consciousness. Do not rely solely on your therapy for your arthritis management, and do not replace or stop your conventional treatment without your doctor's approval. Use your therapy as a complement or an alternative to your conventional treatment, and maintain a balanced and healthy lifestyle. Follow your doctor's recommendations for your medication, exercise, diet, and self-care.

Ways to Combine and Integrate Different Therapies for Optimal Results

You can combine and integrate different complementary and alternative therapies for your arthritis management, as long as they are compatible and safe for you, and do not interfere with your conventional treatment. Some examples of possible combinations and integrations are:

- **Acupuncture and massage**: You can use acupuncture and massage together to enhance the pain relief and relaxation effects of both therapies. Acupuncture can stimulate the nerves and release endorphins, while massage can relax the muscles and improve the blood flow. You can have acupuncture and massage sessions on the same day or on different days, depending on your schedule and preference.

- **Yoga and meditation**: You can use yoga and meditation together to improve the physical and mental aspects of your arthritis management. Yoga can strengthen, balance, and stretch your joints, while meditation can calm, focus, and cope with your mind. You can practice yoga and meditation in the same session or in separate sessions, depending on your time and mood.

- **Aromatherapy and music therapy**: You can use aromatherapy and music therapy together to enhance the mood and sleep effects of both therapies. Aromatherapy can stimulate the senses and release serotonin, while music therapy can soothe the emotions and regulate the brain waves. You can use aromatherapy and music therapy in the same room or in different rooms, depending on your space and comfort.

- **Probiotics and ginger**: You can use probiotics and ginger together to improve the immune and digestive effects of both therapies. Probiotics can balance the gut flora and boost the natural defenses, while ginger can reduce the inflammation and nausea. You can take probiotics and ginger in the same meal or in different meals, depending on your taste and appetite.

- **Glucosamine and chondroitin and omega-3 fatty acids**: You can use glucosamine and chondroitin and omega-3 fatty acids together to improve the joint and cartilage effects of both therapies. Glucosamine and chondroitin can slow down the degeneration and repair the damage of the cartilage, while omega-3 fatty acids can reduce the inflammation and lubricate the joints. You can take glucosamine and chondroitin and omega-3 fatty acids in the same capsule or in different capsules, depending on your convenience and availability.

Complementary and alternative therapies can offer various benefits for people with arthritis, such as reducing pain, inflammation, and stiffness, improving joint function and flexibility, relieving stress and anxiety, boosting mood and energy, and supporting overall health and immunity. However, they are not a substitute for conventional medicine, and they should be used with caution and guidance from your doctor and therapist.

Chapter 6: Managing Your Stress and Emotions for Arthritis

Living with arthritis can be challenging, not only physically, but also emotionally and psychologically. Arthritis can affect your mood, self-esteem, relationships, work, and leisure activities. You may experience stress, anxiety, depression, anger, frustration, or guilt as a result of your condition. These negative emotions can worsen your pain, inflammation, and disability, creating a vicious cycle that is hard to break.

However, you are not alone in this struggle. Many people with arthritis face similar challenges and have learned to cope with them effectively. In this chapter, we will explore some of the common emotional and psychological issues that arise from living with arthritis, and how you can manage them with various strategies and techniques. We will also discuss the benefits of relaxation and how to practice it regularly to reduce your stress and improve your well-being. By the end of this chapter, you will have a better understanding of how to deal with your stress and emotions for arthritis, and how to cultivate a positive mindset that will help you live a fulfilling and satisfying life.

The Emotional and Psychological Challenges of Living with Arthritis

Arthritis can affect your emotional and psychological health in many ways. Some of the common challenges that people with arthritis face are:

- **Stress**: Stress is a natural response to any threat or challenge that you encounter. It can help you cope with difficult situations and motivate you to take action. However, too much stress can be harmful to your health and well-being. Stress can trigger or worsen inflammation, pain, and fatigue in people with arthritis. It can also impair your immune system, making you more susceptible to infections and other illnesses. Stress can also affect your mood, behavior, and cognition, leading to irritability, anxiety, poor concentration, and memory problems.

- **Anxiety**: Anxiety is a feeling of fear, nervousness, or worry about something that may or may not happen in the future. It can also cause physical symptoms such as racing heart, sweating, trembling, shortness of breath, and nausea. Anxiety can interfere with your daily activities and quality of life. People with arthritis may experience anxiety for various reasons, such as uncertainty about their prognosis, fear of pain or disability, concern about their appearance or social acceptance, or worry about their finances or family responsibilities.

- **Depression**: Depression is a mood disorder that causes persistent sadness, loss of interest, hopelessness, and low self-esteem. It can also affect your appetite, sleep, energy, and motivation. Depression can impair your ability to function normally and enjoy life. People with arthritis may develop depression as a result of their chronic pain, disability, isolation, or loss of identity. Depression can also make your pain and inflammation worse, as well as increase your risk of cardiovascular disease and other complications.

- **Low self-esteem**: Self-esteem is how you value and respect yourself as a person. It affects your confidence, self-worth, and happiness. Low self-esteem can make you feel insecure, inadequate, or unworthy. It can also make you more vulnerable to criticism, rejection, or failure. People with arthritis may have low self-esteem due to their physical limitations, appearance, or perceived lack of competence or productivity. Low self-esteem can also affect your relationships, career, and hobbies, as well as your willingness to seek help or try new things.

- **Anger**: Anger is a normal and healthy emotion that expresses your displeasure or dissatisfaction with something or someone. It can help you assert your rights, defend yourself, or change a situation. However, excessive or inappropriate anger can be harmful to yourself and others. It can damage your relationships, reputation, and health. Anger can also increase your pain, blood pressure, and heart rate. People with arthritis may feel angry about their condition, its impact on their life, or the lack of support or understanding from others. They may also feel angry at themselves, their doctors, or their fate.

These emotional and psychological challenges can be overwhelming and difficult to cope with. However, they are not inevitable or permanent. You can learn to manage and overcome them with the help of various strategies and techniques.

The Strategies and Techniques for Managing and Overcoming Your Stress and Emotions for Arthritis

There are many ways to deal with your stress and emotions for arthritis. Some of the most effective and widely used strategies and techniques are:

1. **Cognitive-behavioral therapy (CBT)**: CBT is a type of psychotherapy that helps you identify and change your negative thoughts, beliefs, and behaviors that contribute to your stress and

emotions. CBT teaches you how to replace your irrational or distorted thoughts with more realistic and positive ones, and how to cope with your emotions in a healthier and more constructive way. CBT can help you reduce your stress, anxiety, depression, anger, and pain, as well as improve your self-esteem, mood, and quality of life. CBT can be delivered by a trained therapist, in individual or group sessions, or through self-help books, online programs, or apps.

2. **Mindfulness**: Mindfulness is a state of awareness and attention to the present moment, without judgment or reaction. Mindfulness can help you cope with your stress and emotions by helping you accept your situation, detach from your thoughts and feelings, and focus on the positive aspects of your life. Mindfulness can also help you reduce your pain, inflammation, and fatigue, as well as enhance your immune system, brain function, and well-being. Mindfulness can be practiced through

various methods, such as meditation, yoga, breathing exercises, or body scans.

3. **Positive affirmations**: Positive affirmations are statements that you repeat to yourself to reinforce your positive qualities, abilities, and goals. Positive affirmations can help you boost your self-esteem, confidence, and optimism, as well as reduce your stress, anxiety, and depression. Positive affirmations can also help you change your negative self-talk and beliefs, and create a more positive and empowering mindset. Positive affirmations can be written, spoken, or listened to, and should be specific, realistic, and meaningful to you. Some examples of positive affirmations for arthritis are:

- I am strong and resilient, and I can overcome any challenge.

- I am grateful for all the things I can do, and I celebrate my achievements.

- I am worthy of love, respect, and happiness, and I have supportive and caring people in my life.

- I am in control of my pain, and I can manage it effectively.

- I am optimistic about my future, and I have exciting and fulfilling goals to pursue.

The Benefits of Relaxation and How to Practice It Regularly

Relaxation is a state of calmness and peace that reduces your physical and mental tension and stress. Relaxation can have many benefits for your health and well-being, such as:

- Reducing your pain, inflammation, and stiffness.
- Lowering your blood pressure, heart rate, and cortisol levels.
- Improving your immune system, digestion, and sleep quality.
- Enhancing your mood, memory, and creativity.
- Increasing your energy, motivation, and productivity

Relaxation can be achieved through various techniques and exercises that involve your body, mind, or both. Some of the most common and effective relaxation techniques and exercises are:

1. **Deep breathing**: Deep breathing is a simple and easy way to relax your body and mind. It involves inhaling deeply through your nose, filling your lungs with air, and exhaling slowly through your mouth, emptying your lungs completely. Deep breathing can help you lower your stress, anxiety, and pain, as well as improve your oxygen intake, blood circulation, and heart function. You can practice deep breathing anytime and anywhere, by following these steps:

- Sit or lie down in a comfortable position, with your back straight and your shoulders relaxed.

- Place one hand on your chest and the other on your abdomen.

- Breathe in slowly and deeply through your nose, feeling your abdomen rise as you inhale.

- Breathe out slowly and gently through your mouth, feeling your abdomen fall as you exhale.

- Repeat this cycle for several minutes, focusing on your breathing and letting go of any thoughts or worries.

2. **Progressive muscle relaxation (PMR)**: PMR is a technique that involves tensing and relaxing different muscle groups in your body, one by one. PMR can help you release your physical tension and stress, as well as reduce your pain, inflammation, and fatigue. It can also help you become more aware of your body and its sensations, and improve your posture and flexibility. You can practice PMR by following these steps:

- Sit or lie down in a comfortable position, with your eyes closed and your breathing normal.

- Start with your feet and toes, and tense them as hard as you can for about 5 seconds, feeling the tension in your muscles.

- Relax your feet and toes, and feel the difference as they become loose and relaxed.

- Move up to your calves, and repeat the same process of tensing and relaxing them for about 5 seconds each.

- Continue with your thighs, buttocks, abdomen, chest, back, arms, hands, neck, face, and head, tensing and relaxing each muscle group for about 5 seconds each.

- When you finish, take a few deep breaths and enjoy the feeling of relaxation throughout your body.

3. **Guided imagery**: Guided imagery is a technique that involves using your imagination to create a vivid and pleasant scene in your mind. Guided imagery can help you relax your mind and body, as well as reduce your stress, anxiety, and pain. It can also help you enhance your mood, creativity, and self-esteem. You can practice guided imagery by following these steps:

- Sit or lie down in a comfortable position, with your eyes closed and your breathing normal.

- Think of a place that makes you feel calm, happy, and safe. It can be a real or imaginary place, such as a beach, a forest, a garden, or a cozy room.

- Use your senses to imagine the details of the scene, such as the colors, sounds, smells, textures, and tastes. For example, if you are imagining a beach, you can see the blue sky and the sparkling water, hear the waves and the seagulls, smell the salt and the sand, feel the sun and the breeze, and taste the coconut and the pineapple.

- Stay in the scene for as long as you like, and enjoy the feeling of relaxation and peace that it brings you.
- When you are ready, gently open your eyes and return to the present moment.

4. **Music therapy**: Music therapy is the use of music to improve your physical, mental, and emotional health. Music can help you relax your body and mind, as well as reduce your stress, anxiety, depression, and pain. It can also help you improve your mood, memory, and cognition, as well as stimulate your creativity and expression. You can practice music therapy by listening to, playing, or singing music that you like, or by following a guided music program designed by a professional music therapist. Some of the benefits of music therapy for arthritis are:

- Listening to soothing music can lower your blood pressure, heart rate, and cortisol levels, as well as increase your endorphins and serotonin levels, which are natural painkillers and mood boosters.

- Listening to upbeat music can energize you, motivate you, and improve your mood and outlook.

- Playing or singing music can distract you from your pain, improve your motor skills and coordination, and enhance your self-confidence and self-expression.

- Following a guided music program can help you cope with your emotions, learn new skills, and achieve your goals.

These are some of the relaxation techniques and exercises that you can try to manage your stress and emotions for arthritis. However, there are many other methods that you can explore and experiment with, such as aromatherapy, massage, acupuncture, biofeedback, hypnosis, art therapy, or journaling. The key is to find what works best for you, and practice it regularly and consistently. Relaxation can have a profound impact on your health and well-being, and can make a positive difference in your life.

The Ways to Cope with Negative Thoughts and Feelings and Cultivate a Positive Mindset

One of the most important aspects of managing your stress and emotions for arthritis is to cope with your negative thoughts and feelings and cultivate a positive mindset. Your thoughts and feelings can influence your behavior, actions, and outcomes, as well as your pain, inflammation, and disability. Therefore, it is essential to learn how to deal with them effectively and constructively, and how to create a more positive and empowering mindset that will help you cope with your condition and improve your quality of life. Some of the ways to do this are:

1. **Challenge your negative thoughts and feelings**: Negative thoughts and feelings are often irrational, exaggerated, or distorted, and do not reflect the reality of your situation. They can also be self-defeating, self-critical, or self-blaming, and can undermine your self-esteem and confidence.

Therefore, it is important to challenge them and replace them with more realistic and positive ones. You can do this by asking yourself questions such as:

- Is this thought or feeling based on facts or assumptions?
- Is this thought or feeling helpful or harmful to me?
- Is there any evidence to support or contradict this thought or feeling?
- What would I say to a friend who had this thought or feeling?
- How can I reframe this thought or feeling in a more positive or constructive way?

For example, if you have the thought "I am useless and worthless because I have arthritis", you can challenge it by asking yourself:

- Is this thought based on facts or assumptions? It is based on assumptions, not facts. Having arthritis does not make me useless or worthless. I have many qualities, skills, and talents that make me valuable and useful.

- Is this thought helpful or harmful to me? It is harmful to me, because it makes me feel bad about myself and lowers my self-esteem and confidence. It also prevents me from pursuing my goals and enjoying my life.

- Is there any evidence to support or contradict this thought? There is no evidence to support this thought, but there is plenty of evidence to contradict it. For example, I have a loving family and friends who care about me and appreciate me. I have a successful career and a fulfilling hobby that I enjoy. I have achieved many things in my life and have overcome many challenges.

- What would I say to a friend who had this thought? I would say that they are not useless or worthless because they have arthritis. I would say that they are strong and resilient, and that they have many positive attributes and abilities that make them valuable and useful. I would say that they have a lot to offer to the world and to themselves, and that they should be proud of who they are and what they have done.

- How can I reframe this thought in a more positive or constructive way? I can reframe this thought by saying "I am valuable and useful, despite having arthritis. I have many qualities, skills, and talents that make me unique and special. I have a lot to contribute to the world and to myself, and I can achieve anything I set my mind to."

2. **Express your negative thoughts and feelings**: Sometimes, the best way to cope with your negative thoughts and feelings is to express them, rather than suppress them or avoid them. Expressing your negative thoughts and feelings can help you release your tension and stress, as well as gain insight and perspective on your situation. It can also help you receive support and feedback from others, who can empathize with you, validate you, or offer you advice or solutions. You can express your negative thoughts and feelings by:

- Talking to someone you trust, such as a family member, friend, therapist, or support group. They can listen to you, understand you, and comfort you, as well as offer you their opinions, suggestions, or experiences.

- Writing them down in a journal, a letter, or a blog. Writing can help you organize your thoughts and feelings, and clarify your problems and goals. It can also help you vent your emotions and release your negativity, as well as track your progress and achievements.

- Creating something artistic, such as a painting, a song, or a poem. Art can help you express your thoughts and feelings in a creative and symbolic way, and communicate them to others or yourself. It can also help you channel your emotions and energy into something positive and productive, as well as enhance your self-esteem and self-expression.

3. **Focus on the positive aspects of your life**: Another way to cope with your negative thoughts and feelings is to focus on the positive aspects of your life, rather than the negative ones. Focusing on the positive aspects of your life can help you balance your perspective and attitude, and appreciate what

you have, rather than what you lack. It can also help you boost your mood, optimism, and gratitude, as well as reduce your stress, anxiety, and depression. You can focus on the positive aspects of your life by:

- Practicing gratitude, which is the act of being thankful for the things, people, and experiences that you have in your life. Gratitude can help you recognize and appreciate the good things in your life, and how they benefit you or make you happy. You can practice gratitude by writing down or saying out loud three things that you are grateful for every day, or by expressing your gratitude to someone who has helped you or made a difference in your life.

- Celebrating your achievements, which are the things that you have accomplished or done well in your life. Celebrating your achievements can help you acknowledge and appreciate your efforts and results, and how they reflect your abilities and potential. You can celebrate your achievements by rewarding yourself with something that you enjoy, such as a treat, a gift, or a compliment, or by sharing your achievements with others, such as your family, friends, or social media.

- Engaging in positive activities, which are the things that you enjoy doing or that make you feel good. Positive activities can help you have fun and pleasure, and enhance your well-being and happiness. You can engage in positive activities by doing something that you love, such as a hobby, a sport, or a leisure activity, or by trying something new, such as a skill, a challenge, or an adventure.

These are some of the ways to cope with your negative thoughts and feelings and cultivate a positive mindset. However, there are many other methods that you can explore and experiment with, such as reading inspirational books, watching motivational videos, listening to uplifting podcasts, or following role models or mentors. The key is to find what works best for you, and practice it regularly and consistently. A positive mindset can have a powerful impact on your health and well-being, and can make a positive difference in your life.

Living with arthritis can be hard, but it does not have to define you or limit you. You can learn to cope with your stress and emotions for arthritis, and improve your quality of life, by applying the strategies and techniques that we have covered in this chapter. Remember that you are not alone in this journey, and that you have the power and the potential to overcome any challenge that you face. You are strong, resilient, and valuable, and you deserve to be happy and healthy.

Arthritis can impact more than just joints; it can also affect organs, such as the heart, lungs, and eyes, particularly in cases of autoimmune arthritis like rheumatoid arthritis.

Chapter 7: Building and Maintaining Your Social Support for Arthritis

Living with arthritis can be challenging, both physically and emotionally. You may experience pain, stiffness, fatigue, and reduced mobility that affect your daily activities and quality of life. You may also face stress, anxiety, depression, and low self-esteem as a result of your condition. That is why having a strong social support network is crucial for your well-being and coping with arthritis.

Social support is the emotional, practical, and informational assistance that you receive from others who care about you and your health. It can help you in many ways, such as:

- Providing comfort, encouragement, and empathy.
- Sharing experiences, advice, and information.
- Offering practical help, such as running errands, doing chores, or driving you to appointments.
- Helping you cope with negative emotions and stress.

- Motivating you to adhere to your treatment plan and adopt healthy behaviors.
- Enhancing your self-esteem and confidence.
- Reducing your sense of isolation and loneliness.
- Improving your mood and mental health

Research has shown that people with arthritis who have higher levels of social support tend to have better outcomes, such as lower pain intensity, less disability, greater physical function, and higher quality of life . Therefore, it is important to build and maintain a social support network that meets your needs and preferences.

Types and Sources of Social Support

There are different types of social support that you may need or want, depending on your situation and personality. These include:

- **Emotional support**: This is the most common and basic type of support, which involves expressing care, concern, sympathy, and affection. It can help you feel loved, valued, and understood, and reduce your emotional distress. Examples of emotional support are listening to your problems, giving you a hug, or telling you that you are not alone.

- **Practical support**: This type of support involves providing tangible help or assistance with tasks that you may have difficulty with due to your arthritis. It can help you manage your daily responsibilities and reduce your physical burden. Examples of practical support are helping you with household chores, shopping, cooking, or driving you to appointments.

- **Informational support**: This type of support involves providing useful information or advice that can help you deal with your arthritis or improve your situation. It can help you learn more about your condition, treatment options, coping strategies, and resources. Examples of informational support are recommending a good doctor, sharing a helpful website, or suggesting a new exercise.

- **Companionship support**: This type of support involves providing social interaction and a sense of belonging. It can help you feel less isolated and lonely, and more connected and engaged with others. Examples of companionship support are inviting you to a social event, joining you for a walk, or calling you for a chat.

You can receive different types of social support from various sources, such as:

- **Family**: Your family members, such as your spouse, children, parents, siblings, or relatives, can be a vital source of support for you. They may know you best and care for you deeply, and they may be able to provide you with emotional, practical, informational, and companionship support. However, they may also have their own challenges and needs, and they may not always understand your condition or how to help you. Therefore, it is important to communicate clearly and respectfully with your family, and express your gratitude and appreciation for their support.

- **Friends**: Your friends, such as your classmates, coworkers, neighbors, or acquaintances, can also be a valuable source of support for you. They may share similar interests, hobbies, or experiences with you, and they may be able to provide you with emotional, practical, informational, and companionship support. However, they may also have their own commitments and obligations, and they may not always be available or reliable. Therefore, it is important to maintain and nurture your friendships, and be supportive and respectful of their needs and boundaries.

- **Peers**: Your peers are people who have arthritis or a similar condition, and who can relate to your challenges and feelings. They can be a unique source of support for you, as they can provide you with emotional, informational, and companionship support. They can also offer you a different perspective, inspire you with their stories, and motivate you with their achievements. You can find your peers through support groups, online forums, or social media platforms, where you can share your experiences, ask questions, and exchange tips and resources.

- **Professionals**: Your professionals are people who have expertise or training in arthritis or related fields, and who can provide you with informational and practical support. They can include your doctors, nurses, pharmacists, physiotherapists, occupational therapists, psychologists, counselors, or coaches. They can help you with your diagnosis, treatment, medication, rehabilitation, pain management, mental health, and lifestyle changes. You can find your professionals through your health care system, community organizations, or online platforms, where you can consult them, seek their advice, or access their services.

- **Online communities**: Online communities are groups of people who interact through the internet, using websites, apps, or social media platforms. They can provide you with emotional, informational, and companionship support, as well as access to a large and diverse network of people who have arthritis or similar conditions. You can join online communities that are specific to your type of arthritis, your location, your age, your gender, or your interests, where you can post messages, read articles, watch videos, or join chats and webinars.

Tips and Strategies for Building and Maintaining a Strong Support Network

Having a strong support network can make a big difference in your life with arthritis, but it may not always be easy to build and maintain one. Here are some tips and strategies that can help you:

- **Identify your needs and preferences**: Before you seek support, it is helpful to identify what type of support you need or want, and from whom. You may need different types of support at different times, depending on your situation and mood. You may also prefer different sources of support, depending on your personality and comfort level.

For example, you may need emotional support from your family, practical support from your friends, informational support from your peers, and companionship support from your online community. Or you may prefer to receive support from people who are close to you, or from people who are anonymous. Knowing your needs and preferences can help you find the right support for you.

- **Reach out and ask for help**: Sometimes, you may hesitate to reach out and ask for help, because you may feel embarrassed, guilty, or burdensome. You may also think that others are too busy, or that they do not care. However, these are often false assumptions, and they can prevent you from getting the support that you need and deserve. Remember that most people are willing and happy to help, if they know how. Therefore, do not be afraid to reach out and ask for help, and be specific and clear about what you need or want. For example, you can say, "I am feeling down today, can you talk to me for a while?" or "I have a doctor's appointment tomorrow, can you drive me there?" or "I am looking for a good exercise program, do you have any recommendations?" By reaching out and asking for help, you are not only getting the support that you need, but also strengthening your relationships and showing your trust and respect for others.

- **Be open and honest**: When you receive support, it is important to be open and honest with your supporters, and let them know how you feel and what you think. This can help them understand your condition and your situation better, and provide you with more appropriate and effective support. It can also help you express your emotions and thoughts, and reduce your stress and frustration. For example, you can say, "I appreciate your help, but I feel like I can do this on my own." or "I know you mean well, but your advice is not very helpful for me." or "I am glad you are here, but I need some time alone." By being open and honest, you are not only getting the support that you want, but also enhancing your communication and intimacy with others.

- **Give and receive feedback**: When you receive support, it is also important to give and receive feedback, and let your supporters know how their support affects you and how they can improve it. This can help them adjust their support to your needs and preferences, and provide you with more satisfying and beneficial support. It can also help you acknowledge their efforts and show your gratitude and appreciation. For example, you can say, "Thank you for listening to me, it really helps me feel better." or "I like your suggestion, I will try it out." or "I appreciate your offer, but I would prefer something else." By giving and receiving feedback, you are not only getting the support that you need, but also encouraging and rewarding your supporters and reinforcing their support.

- **Reciprocate and offer support**: When you receive support, it is also important to reciprocate and offer support, and let your supporters know that you care about them and their health. This can help you balance your relationship and avoid feeling dependent or indebted. It can also help you feel good about yourself and boost your self-esteem and confidence. For example, you can say, "How are you doing today?" or "Do you need any help with anything?" or "I am here for you if you ever need to talk." By reciprocating and offering support, you are not only getting the support that you need, but also giving the support that others need and strengthening your bond and friendship with them.

Examples and Suggestions of How to Communicate and Interact with Your Support Network

Communication and interaction are essential for building and maintaining a strong support network. They can help you express your needs and preferences, receive and provide feedback, share your experiences and emotions, and strengthen your relationships. Here are some examples and suggestions of how to communicate and interact with your support network:

- **Use positive and respectful language**: When you communicate and interact with your supporters, it is important to use positive and respectful language, and avoid negative and aggressive language. This can help you convey your message more clearly and effectively, and prevent misunderstandings and conflicts. For example, you can say, "I appreciate your concern, but I feel like I need some space right now." instead of "Leave me alone, you are annoying me." or "I am sorry to hear that, how can I help you?" instead of "That sucks, what do you want me to do?"

- **Be assertive and confident**: When you communicate and interact with your supporters, it is also important to be assertive and confident, and avoid being passive or aggressive. This can help you express your opinions and feelings, stand up for your rights and needs, and respect those of others. For example, you can say, "I would like to join you for dinner, but I have some dietary restrictions."

instead of "I don't care, whatever you want." or "I have some dietary restrictions, so you have to cook something else for me."

- **Use active listening and empathy**: When you communicate and interact with your supporters, it is also important to use active listening and empathy, and avoid being distracted or judgmental. This can help you show your interest and attention, understand their perspective and emotions, and respond appropriately. For example, you can say, "I can see that you are upset, what happened?" instead of "Why are you crying?" or "That sounds tough, I am sorry you had to go through that." instead of "That's not a big deal, you should get over it."

- **Use humor and fun**: When you communicate and interact with your supporters, it is also important to use humor and fun, and avoid being serious or boring. This can help you lighten the mood, reduce stress, and enhance your enjoyment and satisfaction. For example, you can say, "You look great today, did you do something different?" instead of "You look tired today, are you okay?" or "Let's play a game, I bet I can beat you." instead of "Let's watch TV, there is nothing else to do."

- **Use different modes and methods**: When you communicate and interact with your supporters, it is also important to use different modes and methods, and avoid being monotonous or repetitive. This can help you diversify your communication and interaction, and suit your preferences and availability. For example, you can use phone calls, text messages, emails, video calls, or social media to communicate with your supporters, and you can use cards, gifts, flowers, or gestures to show your appreciation and affection. You can also use different methods to interact with your supporters, such as talking, listening, reading, writing, watching, playing, or doing something together.

Ways to Deal with Isolation and Loneliness and Seek Help When Needed

Even if you have a strong support network, you may still feel isolated and lonely at times, especially if you have arthritis. You may feel that no one understands what you are going through, or that you are a burden to others. You may also feel that you have lost your sense of identity, purpose, or belonging. These feelings can be harmful to your physical and mental health, and they can affect your ability to cope with arthritis.

Therefore, it is important to deal with isolation and loneliness, and seek help when needed. Here are some ways that can help you:

- **Recognize and acknowledge your feelings**: The first step to deal with isolation and loneliness is to recognize and acknowledge your feelings, and not to deny or lignore them. You can do this by writing them down, talking to someone, or expressing them through art or music. This can help you understand the causes and effects of your feelings, and find ways to cope with them.

- **Challenge and change your negative thoughts**: The second step to deal with isolation and loneliness is to challenge and change your negative thoughts, and not to believe or accept them. You can do this by identifying the irrational or distorted thoughts that make you feel isolated and lonely, such as "I am alone", "I am worthless", or "I have nothing to offer". Then, you can replace them with more realistic and positive thoughts, such as "I have people who care about me", "I have value and dignity", or "I have skills and talents". This can help you improve your self-image and outlook, and reduce your emotional distress.

- **Engage and connect with others**: The third step to deal with isolation and loneliness is to engage and connect with others, and not to isolate or withdraw from them. You can do this by reaching out and contacting your existing support network, or by expanding and creating a new one. You can also join activities, groups, or events that interest you, or volunteer for a cause that you care about. This can help you increase your social interaction and involvement, and enhance your sense of belonging and meaning.

- **Seek professional help**: The fourth step to deal with isolation and loneliness is to seek professional help, and not to suffer or cope alone. You can do this by consulting your doctor, therapist, counselor, or coach, who can provide you with appropriate treatment, medication, therapy, or coaching. They can also refer you to other resources or services that can help you. This can help you address the underlying issues and factors that contribute to your isolation and loneliness, and improve your overall health and well-being.

In summary, Social Support and Arthritis Coping

- Identified different types of social support sources: family, friends, peers, professionals, and online communities.
- Strategies for building a strong support network: identifying needs, asking for help, being open,

giving feedback, reciprocating support, using positive language, assertiveness, active listening, humor, and seeking professional help.

- Dealing with isolation and loneliness: recognizing feelings, challenging negative thoughts, engaging with others, and seeking professional help.

- Improving social support can enhance well-being and coping with arthritis.

- Sharing knowledge and skills can help others overcome challenges and enjoy opportunities with arthritis.

Chapter 8: Living Well and Enjoying Life with Arthritis

As previously stated, Arthritis is a chronic condition that affects millions of people around the world. It can cause pain, stiffness, inflammation, and reduced mobility in your joints. Arthritis can also affect your quality of life, your mental health, your relationships, and your ability to do the things you love.

But arthritis does not have to stop you from living well and enjoying life. In fact, there are many ways you can manage your pain and improve your mobility, as well as cope with the emotional and social aspects of living with arthritis. In this chapter, we will share with you some tips and advice on how to live well and enjoy life with arthritis, based on the latest research and the experiences of people who have overcome arthritis and achieved their goals and dreams.

Living well and enjoying life with arthritis is possible, but it requires some adjustments and strategies. Here are some tips and advice that can help you:

- **Follow your treatment plan**. The most important thing you can do to manage your pain and improve your mobility is to follow your treatment plan, as prescribed by your doctor. This may include taking medications, doing physical therapy, applying heat or cold, or using assistive devices. Your treatment plan is designed to reduce your symptoms, prevent further damage, and improve your function. Make sure you follow your doctor's instructions and report any changes or side effects.

- **Exercise regularly**. Exercise is one of the best ways to keep your joints healthy and flexible, as well as to improve your mood, energy, and overall well-being. Exercise can also help you lose weight, which can reduce the pressure on your joints and lower your risk of other health problems. Aim for at least 150 minutes of moderate-intensity aerobic exercise per week, such as walking, swimming, cycling, or dancing. You can also do some strength training, stretching, and balance exercises to improve your muscle strength, range of motion, and stability. Consult your doctor or physical therapist before starting any exercise program and start slowly and gradually. Avoid high-impact or repetitive activities that may worsen your pain or cause injury.

- **Eat a healthy diet**. Eating a healthy diet can help you maintain a healthy weight, reduce inflammation, and provide your body with the nutrients it needs to heal and function. A healthy diet for arthritis should include plenty of fruits, vegetables, whole grains, lean proteins, healthy fats, and water. Avoid foods that may trigger inflammation, such as processed foods, refined sugars, saturated fats, trans fats, and alcohol. Some foods that may have anti-inflammatory properties include fish, nuts, seeds, olive oil, berries, cherries, and green tea. You can also talk to your doctor or nutritionist about taking supplements, such as omega-3 fatty acids, vitamin D, calcium, or glucosamine, to support your joint health and bone density.

- **Manage your stress**. Stress can worsen your pain, inflammation, and mood, as well as affect your immune system and your ability to cope. Stress can also trigger unhealthy behaviors, such as smoking, drinking, overeating, or avoiding activities. Therefore, it is important to manage your stress and find healthy ways to relax and unwind. Some stress management techniques that can help you include deep breathing, meditation, yoga, tai chi, massage, aromatherapy, music, art, or hobbies. You can also seek professional help, such as counseling, therapy, or medication, if you feel overwhelmed or depressed by your stress.

- **Get enough sleep**. Sleep is essential for your body and mind to heal and recharge. Sleep can also affect your pain, inflammation, mood, and energy levels. Lack of sleep can make you more sensitive to pain, more irritable, and less motivated. Therefore, it is important to get enough sleep and follow good sleep hygiene practices. Some tips to improve your sleep quality include sticking to a regular sleep schedule, avoiding caffeine, alcohol, nicotine, and heavy meals before bed, creating a comfortable and dark sleeping environment, using relaxation techniques, such as reading, listening to soothing music, or doing progressive muscle relaxation, to calm your mind and body, and avoiding naps during the day, unless you are very tired or have trouble sleeping at night.

- **Stay positive**. Your attitude and outlook can have a big impact on your pain, mobility, and quality of life. Having a positive attitude can help you cope with the challenges and difficulties of living with arthritis, as well as to appreciate the joys and opportunities that life can offer. A positive attitude can also boost your self-esteem, confidence, and resilience, and inspire you to pursue your goals and dreams. Some ways to cultivate a positive attitude include practicing gratitude, optimism, and humor, focusing on your strengths and achievements, rather than your weaknesses and failures, challenging negative thoughts and beliefs, and replacing them with positive ones, and seeking inspiration and motivation from others, such as role models, mentors, or heroes.

Examples and Stories of People Who Have Overcome Arthritis and Achieved Their Goals and Dreams

One of the best ways to inspire and motivate yourself to live well and enjoy life with arthritis is to learn from the examples and stories of people who have overcome arthritis and achieved their goals and dreams. These are people who have faced the challenges and difficulties of living with arthritis, but have not let them stop them from pursuing their passions and aspirations. They have used their creativity, courage, perseverance, and support to overcome their obstacles and make their dreams come true. Here are some examples and stories of such people:

- **Kristy McPherson**. Kristy McPherson is a professional golfer who has been living with rheumatoid arthritis since she was 11 years old. She was diagnosed after she experienced severe pain and swelling in her knees, ankles, wrists, and fingers. She had to take multiple medications, undergo surgeries, and use crutches and braces to manage her condition. She was told by her doctors that she would never be able to play sports or lead a normal life. But Kristy did not give up on her love for golf. She started playing golf at the age of 15, and found that it helped her cope with her pain and improve her mobility. She also found that golf gave her a sense of purpose, joy, and achievement. She went on to become a successful golfer, winning several tournaments and competing in the LPGA Tour and the Solheim Cup. She also became an advocate and spokesperson for the Arthritis Foundation, raising awareness and funds for arthritis research and education. She says, "Golf has given me so much. It has given me a career, a way to travel the world, and a way to help others. It has also taught me to be strong, positive, and grateful. I don't let arthritis define me. I let golf define me."

- **Nick Vujicic**. Nick Vujicic is a motivational speaker, author, and evangelist who was born with tetra-amelia syndrome, a rare disorder that causes the absence of all four limbs. He also has a form of arthritis that affects his spine and causes him chronic pain. He faced many challenges and hardships growing up, such as bullying, discrimination, depression, and suicidal thoughts. He felt hopeless and worthless, and wondered why he was born this way. But Nick found his faith and his purpose in life, and decided to use his condition as an opportunity to inspire and help others. He started to share his story and his message of hope, love, and faith with the world. He traveled to over 60 countries, spoke to millions of people, and wrote several best-selling books. He also founded a non-profit organization called Life Without Limbs, which provides support and resources for people with disabilities. He also got married, had four children, and learned to do many things that most people would think impossible, such as surfing, swimming, skydiving, and playing soccer. He says, "I don't need arms and legs to be happy. I need a purpose. And I have a purpose. I have a purpose to encourage people, to give them hope, and to show them that God loves them."

- **Maya Angelou**. Maya Angelou was a renowned poet, writer, activist, and teacher who suffered from osteoarthritis for most of her adult life. She developed arthritis in her hips, knees, and hands, which caused her severe pain and limited her mobility. She had to use a cane, a walker, and a wheelchair to get around. She also had to endure several surgeries and injections to ease her symptoms. But Maya did not let arthritis stop her from writing and sharing her voice with the world. She wrote over 30 books, including her famous autobiography, I Know Why the Caged Bird Sings, and her celebrated poem, Still I Rise. She also received many awards and honors, such as the

Presidential Medal of Freedom, the National Medal of Arts, and the Pulitzer Prize nomination. She also taught and mentored many students and young writers, and advocated for civil rights, women's rights, and human rights. She says, "I have learned that I still have a lot to learn. I have learned that people will forget what you said, people will forget what you did, but people will never forget how you made them feel."

Resources and Organizations that Can Help You Live Well and Enjoy Life with Arthritis

Living with arthritis can be challenging and isolating, but you don't have to do it alone. There are many resources and organizations that can help you live well and enjoy life with arthritis, such as the Arthritis Foundation, online forums, and support groups. These resources and organizations can provide you with information, education, guidance, advocacy, and support. They can also connect you with other people who share your experiences, challenges, and goals. Here are some examples of resources and organizations that can help you:

- **The Arthritis Foundation**. The Arthritis Foundation is the largest and most trusted source of information and support for people with arthritis in the United States. The Arthritis Foundation offers a variety of programs and services, such as the Arthritis Resource Finder, the Arthritis Helpline, the Arthritis Today magazine, the Living Your Yes podcast, the Live Yes! Online Community, the Live Yes! Connect Groups, the Live Yes! Arthritis Network, the Live Yes! Events, and the Live Yes! Advocacy. The Arthritis Foundation also funds and supports research, innovation, and advocacy for better treatments and cures for arthritis. You can visit their website at www.arthritis.org or call them at *1-800-283-7800* to learn more and get involved.

- **Online Forums**. Online forums are platforms where you can interact with other people who have arthritis, ask questions, share advice, offer support, and exchange stories. Online forums can help you feel less alone, more informed, and more empowered. You can also learn from the experiences and insights of others who have been through similar situations and challenges. Some examples of online forums for people with arthritis are the Arthritis Foundation's Live Yes! Online Community, the CreakyJoints Online Community, the HealthUnlocked Arthritis Action Network, and the Reddit Arthritis Subreddit. You can join these online forums for free and participate in the discussions, or just browse and read the posts.

- **Support Groups**. Support groups are gatherings of people who have arthritis, where they can meet face-to-face or virtually, and provide each other with emotional, social, and practical support. Support groups can help you cope with the stress, anxiety, and depression that may come with living with arthritis. They can also help you build friendships, confidence, and hope. Support groups can be led by professionals, such as counselors, therapists, or social workers, or by peers, such as fellow arthritis patients or volunteers. Some examples of support groups for people with arthritis are the Arthritis Foundation's Live Yes! Connect Groups, the Arthritis Introspective Support Groups, the American Chronic Pain Association Support Groups, and the Pain Connection Support Groups. You can find a support group near you or online by searching on the websites of these organizations or by asking your doctor or local hospital.

Challenges and Opportunities that Arthritis Can Bring and How to Embrace Them

Arthritis can bring many challenges and difficulties to your life, such as pain, disability, fatigue, isolation, and stigma. These challenges can affect your physical, mental, emotional, and social well-being, and make you feel frustrated, angry, sad, or hopeless. However, arthritis can also bring some opportunities and benefits to your life, such as growth, learning, resilience, compassion, and gratitude. These opportunities can help you discover new strengths, skills, interests, and values, and make you feel empowered, inspired, fulfilled, or happy. The key is to embrace both the challenges and the opportunities that arthritis can bring, and use them to improve yourself and your life. Here are some ways to do that:

- **Accept your condition**. The first step to embrace the challenges and opportunities that arthritis can bring is to accept your condition and its impact on your life. Acceptance does not mean giving up or resigning to your fate. It means acknowledging the reality of your situation, without denying, avoiding, or fighting it. Acceptance can help you reduce your stress, anxiety, and depression, and increase your coping skills, self-efficacy, and well-being. Acceptance can also help you focus on the things you can control, such as your attitude, your actions, and your goals, rather than the things you cannot control, such as your symptoms, your prognosis, and your environment. Acceptance can also help you appreciate the positive aspects of your life, such as your achievements, your relationships, and your opportunities, rather than the negative aspects, such as your limitations, your losses, and your challenges.

- **Adapt to your condition**. The second step to embrace the challenges and opportunities that arthritis can bring is to adapt to your condition and its impact on your life. Adaptation means making changes and adjustments to your lifestyle, your habits, your routines, and your environment, to suit your needs, preferences, and abilities. Adaptation can help you manage your pain and improve your mobility, as well as maintain or enhance your function, productivity, and quality of life. Adaptation can also help you discover new ways of doing things, such as using assistive devices, modifying your home or workplace, or learning new skills. Adaptation can also help you explore new possibilities and opportunities, such as pursuing new hobbies, interests, or careers, or traveling to new places.

- **Challenge yourself**. The third step to embrace the challenges and opportunities that arthritis can bring is to challenge yourself and your condition and its impact on your life. Challenge means setting and pursuing realistic and meaningful goals, overcoming obstacles and difficulties, and achieving success and satisfaction. Challenge can help you improve your physical, mental, emotional, and social well-being, as well as your self-esteem, confidence, and resilience. Challenge can also help you grow and learn from your experiences, such as gaining new knowledge, insights, or perspectives. Challenge can also help you fulfill your potential and realize your dreams, such as reaching your personal, professional, or academic aspirations.

Inspiration and Motivation for You to Live Well and Enjoy Life with Arthritis

The final step to embrace the challenges and opportunities that arthritis can bring is to find inspiration and motivation for you to live well and enjoy life with arthritis. Inspiration and motivation are the forces that drive you to take action, to pursue your goals, and to overcome your difficulties. Inspiration and motivation can come from different sources, such as yourself, others, or the world. Inspiration and motivation can also take different forms, such as words, images, sounds, or feelings. Here are some examples of inspiration and motivation for you to live well and enjoy life with arthritis:

- **Yourself**. You can find inspiration and motivation from yourself, from your own strengths, achievements, values, and dreams. You can inspire and motivate yourself by reminding yourself of how far you have come, how much you have overcome, and how much you have to offer. You can also inspire and motivate yourself by setting and celebrating your own goals, by rewarding yourself for your efforts, and by expressing yourself through your passions and talents. You can also inspire and motivate yourself by creating a positive and supportive self-talk, by affirming your worth and potential, and by challenging your fears and doubts.

- **Others**. You can find inspiration and motivation from others, from the people who love you, support you, and inspire you. You can inspire and motivate yourself by surrounding yourself with positive and encouraging people, such as your family, friends, peers, mentors, or role models. You can also inspire and motivate yourself by seeking and accepting help and advice from others, by joining and participating in communities and groups, and by giving back and helping others. You can also inspire and motivate yourself by learning and following the examples and stories of others who have lived well and enjoyed life with arthritis, such as the ones we shared in this chapter.

- **The world**. You can find inspiration and motivation from the world, from the beauty, wonder, and diversity of nature, culture, and humanity. You can inspire and motivate yourself by exploring and experiencing new things, such as traveling, learning, or trying new activities. You can also inspire and motivate yourself by appreciating and enjoying the simple things, such as the sun, the sky, the flowers, or the music. You can also inspire and motivate yourself by finding and pursuing your purpose, by contributing to a cause or a mission, and by making a positive difference in the world.

Living well and enjoying life with arthritis is not easy, but it is possible. It requires you to accept, adapt, challenge, and inspire yourself, as well as to follow your treatment plan, exercise regularly, eat a healthy diet, manage your stress, get enough sleep, and stay positive. It also requires you to seek and use the resources and organizations that can help you, such as the Arthritis Foundation, online forums, and support groups. And most importantly, it requires you to embrace both the challenges and the opportunities that arthritis can bring, and use them to improve yourself and your life.

I hope that this chapter has provided you with some useful information and practical advice on how to live well and enjoy life with arthritis. I also hope that this chapter has inspired and motivated you to pursue your goals and dreams, and to overcome your difficulties and difficulties. Remember, you are not alone, you are not defined by your condition, and you can live well and enjoy life with arthritis. I believe in you, and I wish you all the best.

Fact:

Genetics, age, joint injury, and obesity are among the risk factors that can contribute to the development of arthritis.

Conclusion

You have reached the end of this book, Arthritis Pain Relief: How to Manage Pain and Improve Mobility. In this book, I share with you some valuable tips and strategies on how to cope with arthritis and live a better life. I also provided you with some useful information and practical advice on how to reduce your pain and improve your mobility, as well as how to deal with the emotional and social aspects of living with arthritis. I also introduced you to some resources and organizations that can help you live well and enjoy life with arthritis, such as the Arthritis Foundation, online forums, and support groups. I have also given you some inspiration and motivation to pursue your goals and dreams and overcome your difficulties.

In summary, this book covers various topics related to arthritis, including obtaining a proper diagnosis, eating well and staying hydrated, exercising and moving more for arthritis, stretching and improving flexibility, using complementary and alternative therapies, managing stress and emotions, building and maintaining social support, and living well and enjoying life with arthritis.

In Chapter 1, I discuss the importance of getting a proper diagnosis, conventional treatments like medications, injections, and surgery, as well as the latest advances in arthritis treatment, such as biologics, stem cells, and gene therapy. They also provide tips and advice on how to ask your doctor and consider factors to consider before starting any treatment. Chapter 2 discusses the role of diet and nutrition in reducing inflammation and pain, sharing the best foods and supplements to eat and avoid for arthritis, as well as the importance of hydration and drinking enough water. They also provide tips for planning and preparing healthy meals and snacks, as well as examples and recipes of arthritis-friendly dishes and drinks.

Chapter 3 discusses the benefits of exercise and physical therapy for strengthening joints and muscles, including the best types and frequency of exercise, tips for safely exercising, and examples of arthritis-friendly exercises and activities. They also provide examples and routines of arthritis-friendly stretches and poses. Chapter 4 discusses the benefits of stretching and improving flexibility for improving range of motion and preventing contractures, as well as the best types and frequencies of stretching. They also provide examples and routines of arthritis-friendly stretches and poses. Chapter 5 defines and scopes complementary and alternative therapies for arthritis, discussing their evidence, research, and effectiveness. They also discuss the most popular and effective therapies for arthritis, such as acupuncture, massage, yoga, meditation, and aromatherapy.

Chapter 6 discusses managing stress and emotions for arthritis, including cognitive-behavioral therapy, mindfulness, positive affirmations, relaxation techniques, and ways to cope with negative thoughts and feelings. Chapter 7 discusses building and maintaining a strong support network, including family, friends, peers, professionals, and online communities. Chapter 8 provides tips and advice for living well and enjoying life with arthritis, including examples and stories of people who have overcome arthritis and introducing resources and organizations like the Arthritis Foundation, online forums, and support groups.

I hope that you have found this book informative, practical, and inspiring. I also hope that you have learned something new and useful from this book. But reading this book is not enough. You need to take action and apply what you have learned. You need to follow your treatment plan, exercise regularly, eat a healthy diet, manage your stress, get enough sleep, and stay positive. You also need to seek and use the resources and organizations that can help you. You also need to accept, adapt, challenge, and inspire yourself, and embrace both the challenges and the opportunities that arthritis can bring. You also need to pursue your goals and dreams, and overcome your difficulties and difficulties.

I know that living with arthritis is not easy, but it is possible. It is possible to live well and enjoy life with arthritis. It is possible to reduce your pain and improve your mobility. It is possible to cope with the emotional and social aspects of living with arthritis. It is possible to discover new strengths, skills, interests, and values. It is possible to grow and learn from your experiences. It is possible to fulfill your potential and realize your dreams.

I believe in you, and I want you to believe in yourself. I want you to take charge of your condition and your life. I want you to live well and enjoy life with arthritis. I hope that this book has been helpful and inspiring for you. I also hope that you will continue to learn and explore more about arthritis and how to cope with it.

Here are some additional resources and references that you can use for further reading and learning:
- The Arthritis Foundation website: www.arthritis.org
- The Arthritis Today magazine: www.arthritistoday.org
- The Living Your Yes podcast: www.arthritis.org/living-with-arthritis/podcasts/living-your-yes.php
- The Live Yes! Online Community:

www.arthritis.org/liveyes

* The Live Yes! Connect Groups: www.arthritis.org/liveyes/connect-groups.php

* The Live Yes! Arthritis Network: www.arthritis.org/liveyes/arthritis-network.php

* The Live Yes! Events: www.arthritis.org/liveyes/events.php

* The Live Yes! Advocacy: www.arthritis.org/liveyes/advocacy.php

* The CreakyJoints Online Community:

* www.creakyjoints.org

* The HealthUnlocked Arthritis Action Network: healthunlocked.com/arthritis-action

* The Reddit Arthritis Subreddit:

- www.reddit.com/r/Thritis

- The Arthritis Introspective Support Groups: www.arthritisintrospective.org

- The American Chronic Pain Association Support Groups: www.theacpa.org

- The Pain Connection Support Groups: www.painconnection.org

Thank you for reading this book. I hope that you have enjoyed it and learned from it. I also hope that you will share it with others who may benefit from it. I would love to hear from you and get your feedback and suggestions. You can contact me through my email at philliprichmond92@gmail.com.

I wish you all the best in your journey to live well.

Special Bonus

Gain access to all my previous and future books.

Please consider writing a review!